1

ADVANCES IN
PEDIATRIC
SPORT
SCIENCES

VOLUME THREE
BIOLOGICAL ISSUES

Oded Bar-Or, MD
McMaster University, Hamilton, Ontario, Canada
Editor

Human Kinetics Books
Champaign, Illinois

Library of Congress Catalog Number: 85-644893
ISBN: 0-87322-204-0
ISSN: 0748-6375

Developmental Editor: Marie Roy
Production Director: Ernie Noa
Copyeditor: Claire Mount
Assistant Editors: Holly Gilly and Phaedra Hise
Typesetter: Brad Colson
Text Layout: Jill Wikgren
Printed By: Braun-Brumfield, Inc.

Printed in the United States of America

10 9 8 7 6 5 4 3 2 1

Human Kinetics Books
A Division of Human Kinetics Publishers, Inc.
Box 5076, Champaign, IL 61825-5076
1-800-DIAL-HKP
1-800-334-3665 (in Illinois)

Contents

About the Series

Advances in Pediatric Sport Sciences, or APSS, is an interdisciplinary series published every other year. Scholarly reviews pertaining to children and physical activity will be reported in each volume, with Volume 1 and each subsequent odd-numbered volume focusing on *biological issues* and Volume 2 and each subsequent even-numbered volume focusing on *behavioral issues*.

Topics covered under biological issues include physiological, biomechanical, medical, and some topics within motor control and development as they pertain to pediatric sport sciences. Behavioral issues will draw upon other topics within motor control and development, sport and exercise psychology, sociology of sport, and anthropology of sport and play.

The series is intended to help advance our understanding of children and their health and well-being as they participate in physical activity. Organized sport, play, and fitness activities are common forms of physical activity that will frequently be considered in the series, but they will not be the only forms considered.

The editor for each volume is selected by the publisher. Persons who may be interested in contributing to the series are encouraged to contact the publisher to learn who the editors are for forthcoming volumes.

Preface

Sport scientists and clinicians have taken a keen interest in recent years in the effects of physical exertion among children. *Advances in Pediatric Sport Sciences*, Vol. 3, provides readers with state-of-the-art reviews on physiological, perceptual, and clinical issues concerning child athletes, pediatric patients, and school-age nonathletes.

The first six chapters examine how growth and maturation affect children's responses to exercise. Gaston Beunen highlights the merits of using biological age as an independent variable in pediatric research and the relevance of biological maturity to physical performance. Anthony Sargeant discusses the little-studied concept of short-term muscle power and its development during growth. Dan M. Cooper also provides a development-oriented review, comparing theoretical predictors with actual data of growth-related changes in the O_2 transport system. Is strength training effective in prepubescents? Does it entail special risk to the child? Arthur Weltman reviews the available answers to these questions. Tony M. Reybrouck analyzes age-related changes in the "anaerobic threshold" and its usefulness for testing children, both healthy and with congenital heart disease. Some responses to exercise can be explained by the way a child perceives the intensity of an effort. Oded Bar-Or and Diane S. Ward review the characteristics of the rating of perceived exertion (RPE) in healthy and sick children and discuss the possibility of using it for exercise prescription.

The final four chapters highlight specific medical issues related to children and exercise. Iron deficiency has often been detected in adult endurance athletes; here Thomas W. Rowland examines its etiology and prevalence among adolescents and suggests guidelines for its management. Bronchial asthma is the most prevalent chronic disease among school-age children. Most patients with asthma, whether or not they are athletically active, will suffer from exercise-induced bronchoconstriction (EIB). H.J. Neijens reviews the possible mechanisms of EIB and the means for its prevention and management. It has been estimated that 140,000 to 350,000 American youths who play sports may have excessive aortic blood pressure—Frederick W. Arensman, James L. Christiansen, and William B. Strong discuss the epidemiology, etiology, and management of juvenile hypertension among child and adolescent athletes. Exercise as a diagnostic tool has been gaining recognition in pediatric cardiology. To complete this volume, David J. Driscoll reviews noninvasive exercise testing of children with congenital cardiac defects or other cardiovascular disorders.

Pediatric sport scientists face a significant challenge in fitting exercise testing methods to children, for whom many of the methods and protocols used with adults are unsuitable. The authors of this volume address relevant advances in methodology and conclude their reviews with "Challenges for Future Research." Although the topics there reflect the author's priorities, they may help direct students and scientists pursuing research in pediatric sport sciences.

1

Biological Age in Pediatric Exercise Research

Gaston Beunen
Institute of Physical Education, Heverlee, Belgium

All those involved in teaching or coaching a group of youngsters are confronted daily with the wide interindividual variability in the physical appearance and characteristics of children of the same chronological age, especially during the pubertal years. As long ago as 1908, Crampton, most probably under the influence of Boas, felt the need for a more realistic criterion than chronological age for the classification of adolescent schoolboys with reference to fitness for participation in athletics programs. At about that time, Pryor (1905) and Rotch (1909) demonstrated that children of the same chronological age showed considerable variability in the degree of ossification of the bones of the hand (Tanner, 1981). This chapter provides an overview of the techniques currently used to assess biological maturity and the relationship between biological maturity and various measures of physical performance, including the maturational characteristics of elite athletes.

BIOLOGICAL MATURITY

Definition and Origins of the Concept

Biological maturation differs in a fundamental way from a measurement of growth such as stature, in that every child completes it by reaching the same endpoint (i.e., becoming fully mature). According to Acheson (1966), *maturation* refers to the successive tissue changes that take place until a final form is achieved. Maturation implies specialization and differentiation of cells, whereas growth is defined as a process involving hyperplasia (increase in cell number), hypertrophy (increase in cell size), and increase in intracellular materials. As pointed out by Falkner and Tanner (1978), the processes of growth and maturation are intimately linked, because differential growth creates form.

Already at the beginning of this century, Crampton (1908), Pryor (1905), and Rotch (1909) recognized the need for a criterion of biological maturity. Since then several techniques have been proposed to assess sexual, skeletal, dental, and morphological maturity (e.g., Acheson, 1966; Falkner, 1958; Kelly & Reynolds, 1947; Marshall, 1978; Milman & Bakwin, 1950; Reynolds & Asakawa, 1951; Roche, 1978; Sawtell, 1929; Todd, 1937). From the available literature on techniques of biological age assessment, we can conclude that a valid criterion of biological maturity must satisfy the following conditions:

- Reflect changes in a biological characteristic
- Reach the same final stage in every individual
- Show a continuous smooth increase, although most often discrete stages on this continuum can be identified
- Be applicable throughout the maturation process
- Be independent of size

Assessment

Table 1.1 presents an overview of the most commonly used measures for the assessment of biological maturity. In assessing sex characteristics, researchers most often use the criteria described by Reynolds and Wines (1948, 1951) and popularized by Tanner (1962). For breast development, pubic hair, and genital development, five discrete stages are clearly described. These stages must be assigned by visual inspection of the nude subject or by taking somatotype photographs and enlarging the specific areas. Recently, findings by Neinstein (1982) suggest that self-assessment of sexual maturation might serve as a noninvasive alternative, but further research is needed in this area. Cross-sectional standards of reference for stages of sex characteristics can be obtained by probit or logit analysis of the boys and girls that show a certain stage at a given age. The percentage of boys or girls that show a certain stage are plotted

Table 1.1   Most Commonly Used Systems and Measures in Assessing Biological Maturity

System	Measure
Sexual maturity	Boys: genital development, pubic hair
	Girls: breast development, pubic hair, age at menarche (retrospective, prospective, status quo)
Morphological maturity	Height age, age at peak height velocity, percentage of adult height
Skeletal maturity	Atlas techniques (Greulich & Pyle, 1959), scoring methods (Roche et al., 1975b; Tanner, Whitehouse, Cameron, et al., 1983; Tanner, Whitehouse, Marshall, et al., 1975)
Dental maturity	Number of emerged teeth; ossification of teeth (Demirjian et al., 1973)

against chronological age, and an algebraic function is then fitted to the observed points (Finney, 1952). Naturally, the ratings can be assigned with much more accuracy if the longitudinal data of a child are available. Such longitudinal standards were prepared by Marshall and Tanner (1969, 1970).

Age at menarche, defined as the first menstrual flow, can be determined retrospectively by interrogating a representative sample of women. The estimated age is then, of course, influenced by error in recall. Among adults restudied after 19 years, Damon, Damon, Reed, and Valadian (1969) found a mean difference of 0.17 ± 0.11 years between actual and recalled age at menarche, whereas in another survey of women restudied after 39 years, Damon and Bajema (1974) noted a mean difference of 0.29 ± 0.09 years between recalled and actual age at menarche. This suggests that the technique is reasonably accurate for group comparisons. The information obtained in a longitudinal or prospective survey would be more accurate, but here other problems inherent to longitudinal research are encountered. Another possibility is to interrogate representative samples of girls who are expected to have experienced menarche and record whether or not periods have started at the time of investigation. Reference standards are constructed from such studies as described for the stages of other sex characteristics, using probits or logits.

For all sexual criteria thus far discussed, the main problem is that the changes that occur are limited to the adolescence period. (In this chapter *adolescence* refers to the period from the first changes in sexual characteristics until adult stature is reached; it thus includes the pubertal period.) Furthermore, the stages are fairly crude, discrete milestones in a continuous process.

Height age and even weight age have been used to estimate morphological age. These developmental ages can easily be found by determining the age at which the given child's actual stature equals the height of the average child. However, the measure has limited usefulness, as it confounds maturity with size. In longitudinal studies, age at peak height velocity is another very useful criterion, but is has the inconvenience of having to follow children over several years at regular intervals to define this pubertal event accurately. An alternative technique is to estimate the percentage of adult height. This technique requires the knowledge of adult height, which can be predicted. The four most common predictors are actual height, chronological age, parental height, and an estimation of biological age—usually skeletal age. The three major techniques are those reported by Bayley (1946); Bayley and Pinneau (1952); Roche, Wainer, and Thissen (1975a); Tanner et al. (1983); and Tanner, Whitehouse, Marshall, Healy, and Goldstein, (1975). Recently, excellent overviews of these techniques and their accuracy and limitations were given by Roche (1984) and Tanner et al. (1983).

Although several attempts have been made to construct a shape development criterion, no useful technique has emerged. According to Goldstein (1984), the technique developed by Bookstein (1978), with particular reference to cephalometrics rather than body shape, opens up a new perspective.

Dental age has usually been estimated from the age of eruption of deciduous and permanent teeth, or from the number of teeth present at a certain age (Demirjian, 1978). Eruption is only one event in the ossification process of the tooth. Moreover, it has no real biological meaning and is disturbed by exogenous factors. For this reason, Demirjian, Goldstein, and Tanner (1973) constructed scales for the assessment of dental maturity. The construction of these scales is based on the same principles as the Tanner-Whitehouse technique (Tanner et al., 1975) for assessing skeletal maturity of the hand and wrist. In 1976 the technique was slightly modified and the sample extended to include 2,047 boys and 2,349 girls (Demirjian & Goldstein, 1976). In the view of Roche, Wainer, and Thissen (1975b), there are difficulties in using dental maturation as a measure of biological age that is meaningful for the whole organism. All other biological age scales show that girls are more advanced than boys within a given chronological age group. However, there are no significant sex differences in the timing of deciduous dental development. The permanent teeth nevertheless erupt slightly earlier in girls, but the differences vary among teeth (Demirjian, 1978).

Skeletal maturity is probably the most commonly used criterion in the assessment of biological age. What is more, it is the best single criterion (Acheson, 1966; Falkner, 1958; Tanner, 1962). Because calcified cartilage and bone are radio-opaque, they can be seen on radiographs taken from a specific area of the human body. The radiographic appearance used to assess skeletal maturity is called a *maturity indicator*. Such an indicator must be present in each child and must appear in a fixed sequence (Roche et al., 1975b). Although there are differences in the skeletal maturation of different parts of the body, the hand and wrist area is the most valuable area for the assessment in the age range from 7 to adulthood. The knee is the area of choice from birth to 6 years because more information is contained in the changes that take place in this area during this period (Roche, 1980). Bilateral assessments are unnecessary because the differences involved are small and not of particular importance.

The main techniques that are widely used in assessing skeletal maturity are the atlas technique (Greulich & Pyle, 1950, 1959) and the scoring or bone-specific-approach techniques of Tanner, Whitehouse, Cameron, et al. (1983), Tanner, Whitehouse, Marshall et al. (1975), and Roche et al. (1975b).

The best and most extensively used standard radiographs that have been published for the hand and wrist are those of Greulich and Pyle (1959). In the atlas method, a given radiograph is compared with a set of standard radiographs taken at ages ranging from birth to maturity. Standards are given separately for each sex for every 3-month interval from birth to 2 years, thereafter for every 6-month interval until 5 years, and then annually until puberty, during which the standards are given semiannually. In the judgment of Roche (1980), the only correct estimation of the skeletal age by this method should be done by assigning separate ages to individual bones and by combining these ages so as to obtain an overall mean age. The most serious drawback to this method is the absence of a maturity scale of its own. Moreover, the sample on which the standards are based is from a high socioeconomic level, resulting in a rate of skeletal maturation that is too rapid for children of average socioeconomic level or from most other countries (Acheson, 1966).

The bone-specific approach was introduced by Acheson (1954) for the hip region. Tanner and Whitehouse (1959) and Tanner, Whitehouse, and Healy (1962) developed a system (TW1) for the hand and wrist. Their system was revised in 1975 (TW2; Tanner et al., 1975). In the TW2 method, either seven or eight maturity stages, depending on the particular bone, are identified and carefully described and illustrated. These maturity stages reflect the distance the individual has traveled along the road from complete immaturity to complete maturity. The chief concern of the authors was to construct a maturity scale. In their view, this scale should be defined in a manner that does not refer directly to age. The scores allotted to the different stages of the different bones were defined in such a way as to minimize the overall disagreement between the different bones. In combining the scores of different bones, Tanner et al. (1975) decided to assign a biological weight to the bones. These weightings were based on the assumptions that the maturation rate of the rays in fingers are very similar and that the maturation of the carpals is probably controlled by different mechanisms from the maturation of the radius-ulna and short bones. The authors also developed a separate scoring system on the same principles for the radius-ulna and short bones (RUS-score) and for the carpals (Carpal-score). Standards for skeletal age were then constructed for the British population. In assigning a given stage to a bone, one should carefully follow the written descriptions provided by the authors. To obtain the skeletal age of an individual, the stages should be converted into maturity scores. The latter are then added up, and this sum is transferred to skeletal age. Taranger et al. (1976) used the Tanner-Whitehouse stages to construct a new system based on the calculation of the mean appearance times of the bone stages.

The Roche-Wainer-Thissen (RWT) method was developed for the assessment of antero-posterior radiographs of the knee (Roche et al., 1975b). The method relies on the use of maturity indicators. After retrieving all the possible maturity indicators for the knee reported in the literature, the authors of this method proceeded to grade these indicators. Thereafter, Roche et al. (1975b) selected those indicators that could be defined with a high degree of reliability. Furthermore, they checked the ability of an indicator to discriminate between children, as well as the universality, validity, and completeness of each indicator. On the basis of these criteria, they selected 34 maturity indicators for the femur, tibia, and fibula. The parameters used to construct the RWT scale are the chronological age at which each indicator is present in 50% of the children in the population sample and the rate of change in each indicator's prevalence with age. These parameters are combined to give a single continuous index, using latent trait analysis. This method made it possible to estimate the sampling error, the statistic of which can only be calculated with the RWT technique. After the grades have been recorded for each bone, they are transferred to a computer program that provides the appropriate skeletal age together with the standard error of estimate.

Interrelationships Among Measures of Biological Maturity

Dental age and skeletal maturity are substantially independent of one another (Demirjian, 1978). Because these two maturity indicators have different embryological origins, with possible differences in genetic control, this seems not too surprising. Skeletal age is closely related to the percentage of adult stature, which led to the establishment of equations for the prediction of adult height (Bayley, 1946; Bayley & Pinneau, 1952; Roche et al., 1975a; Tanner et al., 1975).

From the extensive studies of Nicolson and Hanley (1953); Marshall (1974); Anderson, Thompson, and Popovich (1975); Bielicki (1975); and Bielicki, Knoiarek, and Malina (1984), it became apparent that the indexes of sexual maturation, the ages at which various percentages of adult height are attained, the ages at which different stages of skeletal maturity are attained, and the age of peak height velocity are fairly closely interrelated. This interrelationship is reflected by the fact that, in principal component or factor analytic studies, a first component is extracted on which all indexes load highly, indicating a strong general maturity factor (Bielicki, 1975; Bielicki et al., 1984; Nicolson & Hanley, 1953). In boys as well as girls, Bielicki and co-workers identified a second component that is apparently related to the rate of skeletal maturation during preadolescence. The interrelationships between the maturity character-istics, however, are not strong enough to allow individual predictions from one maturity indicator to another. No single system provides a complete description of the maturation of an individual child. The interrelationships described are, nevertheless, strong enough to indicate the developmental level of a group of children or populations (Malina, 1978a).

BIOLOGICAL MATURITY AND PHYSICAL PERFORMANCE

Physical fitness, like health, is a general concept that can be viewed in many ways. Generally, a distinction is made between the motor and the organic components of fitness. The motor component refers to the neuromuscular movement abilities, whereas the organic component refers to the processes of energy production, transport, and work output.

Mainly in the wake of research in the U.S., numerous test batteries have been proposed and are currently used. In Europe, the *Eurofit test battery* has recently been approved, and its adoption will now be promoted in the countries of the European Council (Comité pour le Dévelopment du Sport [CDS], 1987). Before discussing the relationship between physical performance and maturity, I think it's appropriate to review briefly the relationship between anthropometric characteristics and maturity. Maturity and body size are, indeed, confounded with reference to their effects on performance (Malina, 1975), and an elucidation of the relationship between the two would lead to a better understanding of that between performance and maturity.

Anthropometric Characteristics

When the association between biological maturation and anthropometric characteristics is investigated in a given population, it is often approached in two different ways: by conducting a correlational analysis or by contrasting maturity groups. Both approaches generally lead to the same conclusions.

As already mentioned, skeletal maturity is used in the three major techniques of predicting adult stature (Bayley, 1946; Bayley & Pinneau, 1952; Roche et al., 1975a; Tanner, Whitehouse, Cameron et al., 1983, Tanner, Whitehouse, Marshall et al., 1975), which means that children who are advanced in skeletal maturation are closer to adult stature. Indeed, the coefficient of determination (R^2) between skeletal maturity and the attained percentage of adult stature vary between .605 and .792 in 12- to 17-year-old boys and between .401 and .757 in 10- to 16-year-old girls (Bayley, 1943b; Simmons, 1944). In addition, age at menarche is related to height and height increments, which has led some authors to predict age at menarche from height and weight (Frish, 1974) or from height increments (Ellison, 1981).

Table 1.2 summarizes the correlations between skeletal age and a number of anthropometric dimensions obtained in different studies. Considering that different measurement techniques were used and that the samples stem from

Table 1.2   Correlations Between Skeletal Age and Anthropometric Dimensions in Boys From Three Different Studies

Anthropometric dimension	Chronological age				
	12	13	14	15	16
Height					
Bayley (1943a, 1943b)[b]		.66	.59-.64[a]	.40-.46	.15-.35
Clarke (1971)[c]	.59	.72	.76	.66	.45
Beunen et al. (1978)[d]	.60	.68	.70	.62	.40
Sitting height					
Bayley (1943a, 1943b)		.86	.85-.89	.84-.89	.82-.84
Clarke (1971)	.59	.73	.77	.70	.64
Beunen et al. (1978)	.52	.66	.73	.69	.58
Weight					
Bayley (1943a, 1943b)	.65	.75	.81-.87	.78-.83	.76-.81
Clarke (1971)	.65	.74	.77	.69	.60
Beunen et al. (1978)	.57	.62	.65	.63	.52
Chest circumference					
Bayley (1943a, 1943b)		.66	.72-.81	.71-.74	.64-.65
Clarke (1971)	.57	.72	.76	.71	.58
Beunen et al. (1978)	.49	.56	.62	.62	.52
Calf circumference					
Clarke (1971)	.31	.67	.41	.53	.46
Beunen et al. (1978)	.51	.50	.50	.49	.37
Thigh circumference					
Clarke (1971)	.55	.59	.61	.60	.54
Beunen et al. (1978)	.46	.43	.50	.50	.46

[a]Two coefficients are given because boys were measured at half-yearly intervals. [b]N varies between 34 and 72. [c]$N = 62$. [d]N varies between 528 and 2,829.

different populations, some of them studied more than 30 years apart, we see that the similarities in the correlations are indeed striking. Height and sitting height show the highest correlations at all ages until 14 years. Body weight is also highly correlated, whereas circumferences show somewhat lower correlations. In all three studies, the correlations increase until 14 years of age and thereafter decrease for all measurements.

In girls, as in boys, height is most closely related to skeletal maturity, followed by weight, widths, and circumferences (see Figure 1.1). However, in girls the correlations reach a maximum at about 11 years of age. It follows that in both sexes the highest correlations between skeletal age and anthropometric dimensions are found around the time of peak height velocity.

When maturity groups are contrasted, these associations are also apparent (see Figures 1.2 and 1.3). In Figure 1.2 the mean somatic characteristics of retarded (in maturity) 14-year-old boys with mean skeletal ages of 10 ($n = 192$)

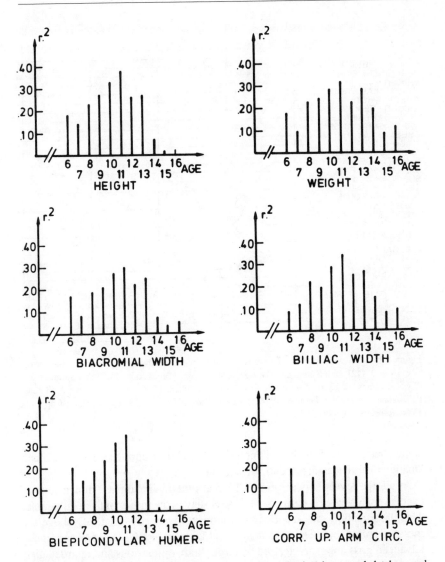

Figure 1.1 Age-specific relationships (coefficients of determination) between skeletal age and selected anthropometric dimensions (*N* varies between 190 and 871). *Note*. From Beunen et al., 1988.

and 11 years (*n* = 622) and of advanced 14-year-old boys with mean skeletal ages of 13 (*n* = 987) and 14 years (*n* = 611) are plotted against the reference values of a national sample of 14-year-old boys (Beunen et al., 1974). The mean height of the most retarded groups (skeletal age = 12 years) is more than 2 SDs removed from the mean height of the most advanced group (skeletal age = 16 years). This implies that more than 68% of the total sample of 14-year-old boys is situated between these two means. The differences decrease

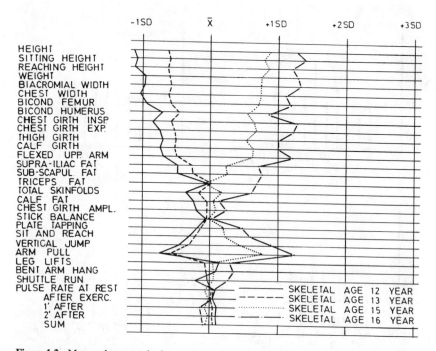

Figure 1.2 Mean anthropometric characteristics of retarded and advanced (in maturity) 14-year-old boys (*N* = 2,412) compared to nationwide reference data. *Note.* From "Skeletal Maturation and Physical Fitness of 12 to 15 Year Old Boys" by G. Beunen, M. Ostyn, R. Renson, J. Simons, P. Swalus, and D. Van Gerven, 1974. *Acta Paediatrica Belgica,* **28**, pp. 221-232. Copyright 1974. Reprinted by permission.

somewhat for trunk widths, bone breadths, and circumferences, and much smaller differences are found for skinfolds.

At all age levels between 6 and 16 years the mean somatic dimensions of average-maturing girls correspond quite closely to the means of the total sample. The classification into groups is as follows: advanced—+1.0 SD above the mean; average—between −0.5 and +0.5 SD; late——1.0 SD. At all age levels, advanced girls are characterized by larger body dimensions and retarded girls by smaller dimensions. The differences are somewhat smaller at the younger ages, increase until puberty, and tend to disappear at 16 years of age, although even at age 16 years, retarded girls still have somewhat lower weight and smaller trunk widths and fat-corrected upper arm circumferences. These trends in the correlations and differences between maturity groups are in close agreement with the findings of Anderson, Hwang, and Green (1965); Bayley (1943a); Beunen, Ostyn, Renson, Simons, and Van Gerven (1976); Beunen, Ostyn, Simons, Renson, and Van Gerven (1981); Beunen et al., (1978); Clarke (1971); Hewitt and Acheson (1961); Johnston (1964); Low, Chan, Chang, and Lee (1968); and Tiisala, Kantero, and Tamminen (1971). The decrease in the relationships after puberty might be accounted for by the greater homogeneity

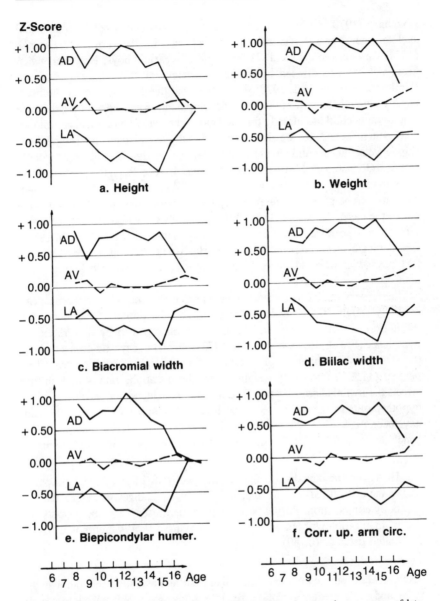

Figure 1.3 Age-specific mean anthropometric characteristics, expressed as z-scores, of late-(LA), average-(AV), and advanced-(AD) maturing girls (*N* varies between 190 and 871) aged between 6 and 16 years. *Note*. From Beunen et al., 1988.

for the different somatic dimensions and by the fact that upon reaching adulthood, each boy and girl attains his or her maximum skeletal maturation.

It has also been demonstrated that heart volume is quite closely related to skeletal age. In a sample of 275 boys, 8 through 18 years old, Hollmann and

Bouchard (1970) observed a correlation of .89 between heart volume and skeletal age. Age-specific correlations reported by Pařízková and Čermák (1977) vary between .12 and .71 for 11- to 18-year-old boys. However, when heart volume was divided by weight, a correlation of −.13 was observed (Hollmann & Bouchard, 1970), indicating that the development of the heart closely parallels total morphological development, irrespective of the distance that a young child has already traveled along the way to biological adulthood.

Muscle mass and size are also associated with skeletal maturity. The relationship is weak during childhood but moderately strong during puberty, especially in boys (Johnston & Malina, 1966; Malina, 1978b; Reynolds, 1946).

As long ago as 1937 Richey demonstrated that, already at 6 years of age, early-menarche girls are characterized by a superior height and weight, long before the menarche occurs. These differences between early- and late-menarche girls are also seen for chest width and bi-iliac diameters (Shuttleworth, 1937). Clark and Degutis (1962) and Clarke and Harrison (1962) further demonstrated that boys who were advanced in pubescent development had higher mean anthropometric dimensions.

Much discussion has centered around a proposed association between a critical body weight (Frisch & Revelle, 1970) and the timing of the menarche, the notion of critical body weight having been replaced by the critical fat hypothesis (Frisch, Revelle, & Cook 1973). The latter investigators advanced the idea that the attainment of a certain critical weight (47 kg) or critical fat percent (17% of total body weight) alters the metabolic rate, which in turn affects the hypothalamic-ovarian feedback loop, reducing the sensitivity of the hypothalamus to circulating estrogen levels. A number of severe criticisms have been made of these hypotheses. After considering these, Malina (1978a) concluded that the critical weight or fat hypothesis was not disproved:

> However, the data do not support the specificity of weight or fatness as the critical variable for menarche. Rather, changes in weight and body compositions during puberty are a manifestation of the process of maturation without either of them having a level which could be called critical. (p. 89)

Obese children not only are fatter than their age and sex peers but also are taller and have greater skeletal size, lean body mass, and muscle mass. In contrast, lean children are correspondingly smaller and retarded in maturity status (Beunen, Malina, et al., 1982; Beunen et al., 1983; Cheek, Schultz, Parra, and Reba, 1970; Garn, Cheek, & Guire, 1975; Garn & Haskell, 1959, 1960; Pařízková, 1977; Quaade, 1955; Seltzer & Mayer, 1964; Wolff, 1955). Correlations between relative skeletal age (skeletal age minus chronological age) and the sum of four skinfolds decreased from $r = .24$ to $r = .13$ in a sample of 14,259 Belgian boys 12 through 17 years of age (Beunen, Malina, et al., 1982). In Flemish 8- to 16-year-old girls the correlations varied from $r = .19$ to $r = .30$ (Beunen et al., 1988).

Early maturers are not only persons whose growth is advanced at all ages; they are also persons who as adults have more weight for height than late maturers (Tanner, 1962). From several studies it can be concluded that in boys the somatotype and its components show a minor relationship to several maturity criteria. In childhood and at the onset of puberty, endomorphy is positively related to skeletal maturity and the age of appearance of pubic hair and genital development (Beunen, 1973-1974; Borms, Hebbelinck, & Ross, 1973; Borms, Hebbelinck, & Van Gheluwe, 1977; Clarke, 1971; Hunt, Cocke, & Gallagher, 1958). Tanner (1962) found no association between endomorphy and the appearance of pubic hair.

Around the age of the growth spurt in height, there is no association between endomorphy and this maturity event (Beunen et al., 1987; Dupertuis & Michael, 1953), and nonsignificant or low positive correlations are found with sex characteristics or skeletal age from 14 through 16 years of age (Beunen, 1973-1974; Clarke, 1971; Hunt et al., 1958). For the period from childhood to early puberty, conflicting results are reported concerning the relationship between mesomorphy and biological maturity. Dupertuis and Michael (1953) observed no differences between mesomorphs and ectomorphs at the onset of the pubertal spurt. With reference to the first appearance of pubic hair, Tanner (1962) noted a decrease in mesomorphy from early to late developers. Skeletal age was positively related to mesomorphy from 10 years of age on in Medford boys (Clarke, 1971). Borms et al. (1973) found no correlations with skeletal age for 10- to 13-year-old boys, whereas Beunen (1973-1974) observed a slight negative correlation at 12 and 13 years of age. After this period, the data reported in the literature consistently point to a small positive correlation between several maturity criteria and the mesomorphy component. Ectomorphs show a tendency to late maturation from the beginning of the pubertal period, although the associations are not statistically significant at all ages (Beunen, 1973-1974; Borms et al., 1977; Dupertuis & Michael, 1953). We may thus conclude that there is a slight association between biological maturation and somatotype. It should be stressed, however, that the chronology of adolescence shows considerable independence of physique as expressed by the somatotype (Barton & Hunt, 1962). In girls, the association between somatotype and maturity has not been carefully investigated. However, late-maturing girls have, on the average, long legs for their stature, relatively narrow hips, less weight for height, and a generally linear physique (Tanner, 1962).

Physical Fitness Components

Maximal Oxygen Uptake.   In analyzing the relationship between physical performance capacity and the criteria of biological age, I make a distinction between associations found in a general population and associations observed in athletes and elite athletes.

First, the association with cardiorespiratory fitness is considered. In a sample of 275 boys 8 to 18 years of age, Hollmann and Bouchard (1970) found a correlation of .887 between skeletal age and maximal oxygen uptake ($\dot{V}O_2$max). At all age levels, significant differences were found between retarded and advanced boys. Smaller coefficients were noted for a group of 8- to 14-year-old trained and untrained children, the correlations having varied between .55 for trained girls and .68 for untrained girls (Labitzke, 1971). It must be pointed out that the age range was much smaller in the 8- to 14-year-old group than in the 8- to 18-year-old group and, moreover, especially in boys, considerable change in $\dot{V}O_2$max still occurs after 14 years of age. When $\dot{V}O_2$max was expressed per kilogram body weight no significant differences were found between maturity groups in 8- to 18-year-old German boys (Hollmann & Bouchard, 1970), 4- to 12-year-old Canadian boys and girls (Shephard et al., 1978), and 11-year-old Bulgarian youngsters (Savov, 1978).

Submaximal Performance Capacity. Correlations between submaximal working capacity and skeletal age for boys are summarized in Table 1.3. Within a given age group, nonsignificant or rather low correlations are found, except around puberty, when substantially higher associations are reported. Bouchard, Leblanc, Malina, and Hollman (1978) pointed out that, in spite of the high degree of relationship between skeletal age, chronological age, height, and weight, a higher association between skeletal age and submaximal working capacity was observed around puberty, although little was added by skeletal age alone. In this investigation, age-specific correlations between skeletal age and submaximal working capacity in girls generally increased with age and reached a maximum at 11 to 13 years of age (see Figure 1.4). The highest

Table 1.3 Correlations Between Skeletal Age and Submaximal Working Capacity in Boys From Different Studies

Author	Sample	Age range (years)	Variable	Bi-variate correlation
Hebbelinck, Borms, & Clarys (1971)	41 Belgian	10 -12.75	PWC170	.37
Kemper et al. (1975)	70 Dutch	11.9-13.7	PWC170	− .12
Bouchard, Malina, Hollmann, & Leblanc (1976)	237 German	8 -18	PWC130 $\dot{V}O_2$130	.764 .795
Bouchard, Leblanc, Malina, & Hollmann (1978)	77 German	8 -11	$\dot{V}O_2$130	.38
	118 German	12 -16	$\dot{V}O_2$130	.68
	42 German	17 -18	$\dot{V}O_2$130	.11

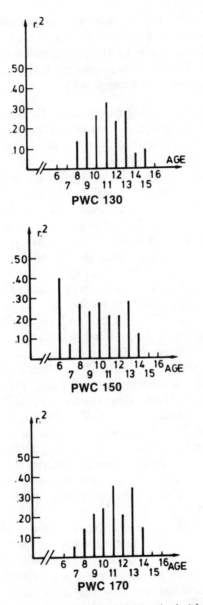

Figure 1.4 Age-specific relationships (coefficient of determination) between skeletal age and submaximal working capacity (*N* varies between 190 and 871). *Note*. From Beunen et al., 1988.

correlation (*r* = .59) was observed between skeletal age and physical working capacity 170 (PWC170) for 13-year-old girls. The age trends in the correlations were less clear for PWC150.

Koinzer (1978) and Koinzer, Enderlein, and Herforth (1981) compared early-, late-, and average-maturing boys and girls. At each age level between

10 and 14 years, early-maturing boys had a higher PWC170 than average- and late-maturing boys. In girls the differences were only significant at 10.9 and 11.8 years of age. For $\dot{V}O_2190$, the differences were less pronounced. In both studies, biological age was assessed by means of a body-build developmental index proposed by Wutscherk (1974).

Motor Performance. In 1940 Espenschade had already demonstrated that in pubescent girls, motor performance levels off or declines with increasing skeletal maturity. Treatment of the same data as a function of age of deviation from menarche yields similar results. Pubescent boys continue to show improved motor performance with increasing skeletal age. Jones (1949) studied 183 cases (93 boys and 90 girls) at half-yearly intervals for 6.5 years. In the boys, skeletal age correlated ($r = .50$) with total strength (grip, pull, and thrust) and early maturers performed better than late maturers at all age levels between 11 and 17 years. Early-maturing girls had an average standard score of 50 at 11 years of age, increasing to 55 at age 13, and thereafter declining to 49, whereas late-maturing girls obtained an average score of 45 to 49. Similar differences were found when girls were classified according to age at menarche. Early-maturing girls performed better than average- or late-maturing girls between 11 and 13 years. Thereafter, however, average-maturing girls obtained the best handgrip scores. Between 10 and 16 years of age, early-maturing boys performed better for upper (shoulder extension, elbow extension, wrist extension and flexion, and elbow flexion) and lower (knee extension and hip flexion) body static strength measurement (Carron & Bailey, 1974), and the same holds true for 7- to 13-year-old girls who experience menarche at an early chronological age (Carron, Aitken, & Bailey, 1977). Finally, Bastos and Hegg (1986) demonstrated that in 11- to 17-year-old boys, pubic hair development accounts for a significant part of the total variance in handgrip strength. These relationships between static or isometric strength and various criteria of biological age are further documented in the extensive studies by Clarke based on the Medford boys' growth study (see Clarke, 1971; Clarke & Degutis, 1962; Clarke & Harrison, 1962).

Correlations between different independent gross motor ability and skeletal age factors are summarized in Tables 1.4 through 1.6. For prepubescent children significant associations are observed for static strength, explosive strength, and running speed when a wide age range is considered. When age-specific correlations are calculated, however, only static strength is associated with skeletal age at all age levels. During adolescence, again, only static strength is positively related to skeletal maturity in girls. For muscular endurance, often called *functional strength* or *dynamic strength*, there is even a negative correlation at 11 through 13 years of age. In boys, static strength is positively related to biological age during adolescence. From 14 years on, however, all the gross motor abilities studied within this period are positively correlated with skeletal age. Muscular endurance tests of the upper body and lower trunk are negatively related to skeletal age in 12- and 13-year-old boys. This is not surprising, because in these tests, the subject acts against his own body weight or a part of it. As for static strength, the highest correlations for all motor items are found at 14 or 15 years of age. These findings, based on correlational analyses, are confirmed by studies in which maturity groups are contrasted with respect to physical performance capacity (Beunen et al., 1974; Clarke & Harrison, 1962; Ellis, Carron, & Bailey, 1975; Petrovcic, Medved, & Horvat, 1957; Savov, 1978; see also Figure 1.2).

Several authors, however, point out that, at least in preadolescent children, the strength of the relationship between skeletal age and motor performance capacities declines considerably when height and especially weight is partialled out (Carron & Bailey, 1974; Rarick & Oyster, 1964; Seils, 1951; Shephard et al., 1978), which observation led them to the conclusion that at these age levels skeletal age is not an important predictor of physical performance capacities. Continuing along these lines, Beunen, Ostyn, Renson, Simons, and Van Gerven (1979) and Beunen, Ostyn, et al. (1981) investigated the correlations between skeletal age and motor performance in adolescent boys. At all age

Table 1.4 Correlations Between Skeletal Age and Motor Performance in Prepubescent Boys (B) and Girls (G)

	Grades 1-3[a]		Grade[b]	7- to 11-year-olds[c]		6-year-olds[d]		Girls (age in years)[e]				
	B	G	Boys	B	G	B	G	6	7	8	9	10
Static strength												
Flexion-extension			.35-.60									
Handgrip						.35	.30					
Arm pull								.25	.21	.25	.31	.39
Explosive strength												
Standing broad jump	.27	.56	.25	.54	.62	.16	ns	ns	ns	ns	ns	ns
Softball throw	.42	.38	.48			ns	ns					
Muscular endurance												
Bent-arm hang				.17	ns			ns	ns	−.11	−.19	−.18
Sit-ups				.36	.17	ns	ns					
Running speed												
Dash	.51	.46	.32	.61	.71	.23	ns					
Shuttle run				.48	.56			.19	ns	ns	ns	ns
Speed of limb movement												
Plate tapping								ns	ns	−.11	ns	+.10
Flexibility												
Sit and reach								ns	ns	−.09	−.10	ns

ns = nonsignificant correlation ($p > .05$)

[a]Seils (1951). [b]Rarick & Oyster (1964). [c]Rajic et al. (1979). [d]Hebbelinck et al. (1986). [e]Beunen et al. (1988).

Table 1.5   Correlations Between Skeletal Age and Motor Performance in 11- to 16-Year-Old Girls

Factor	Test	Source	Age (years)					
			11	12	13	14	15	16
Static strength	Arm pull	a		.35	.33	.28	.28	ns
		b	.39	.35	.39	.26	.17	.23
Explosive strength	Vertical jump	a		ns	ns	ns	ns	ns
		b	ns	.11	.08	.07	ns	ns
Muscular endurance	Bent-arm hang	a		−.42	−.20	ns	ns	ns
		b	−.26	−.19	−.13	ns	ns	ns
	Leg lifts	a		ns	ns	ns	ns	ns
		b	−.21	ns	ns	ns	ns	ns
Running speed	Dodge run	a		ns	ns	ns	ns	ns
	Shuttle run	b	.08	ns	ns	ns	ns	ns
Speed of limb movement	Plate tapping	a		ns	ns	ns	ns	ns
		b	ns	.08	.09	ns	ns	ns
Flexibility	Sit and reach	a		ns	ns	ns	ns	ns
		b	ns	ns	ns	ns	ns	ns

Note. Data from: a = Beunen et al. (1976) and b = Beunen et al. (1988). ns = nonsignificant correlation, $p > .05$.

Table 1.6   Correlations Between Skeletal Age and Motor Performance in 12- to 16-Year-Old Adolescent Boys

Factor	Test	Source	Age (years)				
			11	12	13	14	15
Static strength	Extension-flexion	a	ns	ns	.28	.29	ns
			.44	.68	.81	.67	.54
	Arm pull	b	.43	.55	.65	.63	.51
Explosive strength	Standing broad jump	a	ns	ns	.39	.40	ns
	Vertical jump	b	ns	.20	.32	.38	.32
Muscular endurance	Bent-arm hang	b	−.19	−.14	ns	ns	ns
	Leg lifts	b	−.15	−.12	.04	.13	.19
Running speed	Shuttle run	b	ns	ns	.13	.12	.09
Speed of limb movement	Plate tapping	b	ns	.15	.12	.18	.17
Flexibility	Sit and reach	b	ns	.06	.16	.19	.14

Note. Data from: a = Clarke (1971), and b = Beunen et al. (1978). ns = nonsignificant correlation, $p > .05$.

levels between 13 and 17 years, the third-order partial correlations between skeletal age and speed of limb movement, flexibility, explosive strength, and static strength, with age, height, and weight held constant, were lower than the zero-order coefficients. The third-order coefficients, however, were higher for muscular endurance of upper body and lower trunk and for running speed. All third-order correlations were significant. This implies that 13- to 17-year-old boys advanced in skeletal maturity and of the same chronological age, height, and weight perform better than their less mature peers for all gross motor items. In considering the relative importance of chronological age, height, weight, and skeletal age in the explanation of the variance in motor performance, Beunen, Ostyn, et al. (1981) concluded that at each age level between 12 and 19 years, the interaction between chronological age and skeletal age as such, or in combination with height and/or weight, had a higher predictive value than any other single variable except for performance in muscular endurance tests (bent-arm hang and leg lifts). The predictive value of body size (height and weight), skeletal maturity, and chronological age and their interactions was rather low, having varied between 0% and 17%, except for static strength (arm pull), for which the explained variance ranged from 33% to 58%. As for body dimensions, the explained variance reaches a maximum for most tests at 14-15 years of age.

Athletes and Elite Athletes

A number of investigators have studied the relationship between biological age and specific sport skills within specific population samples. Szabó, Doka, Apor, and Somogyvari (1972) demonstrated that early-maturing swimmers had a better performance in the 100-m freestyle. Cumming (1973) and Szabó and Mészáros (1980) found moderate-to-high correlations between performance in track-and-field events and skeletal age in adolescent males and females. Furthermore, in young soccer players, skeletal age is not related to specific soccer skills (Vrijens & Van Cauter, 1985).

In recent years, excellent reviews of the existing data on maturity characteristics in young athletes have been published by Malina (1978c, 1982, 1983, 1984, 1986, 1988) and Malina, Meleski, and Shoup (1982). The following discussion summarizes the available evidence and discusses the sex-specific maturity characteristics of athletes. In considering these characteristics, we should keep in mind that the analysis is immediately beset with a number of difficulties, as pointed out by Malina, Meleski, and Shoup (1982). First, it is not easy to provide an exact definition of an athlete. Second, successful young athletes are a highly selective group, usually in virtue of their skill, but often also with reference to size and physique. The selection may be carried out by the individual concerned and/or by parents and coaches. Furthermore, the variation in biological maturation is associated with differences in size, physique, body composition, and gross motor performance. Finally, there are many other determinants of successful athletic performance.

Tables 1.7-1.10 provide a summary of the maturity characteristics of male and female athletes. Male athletes of different competitive levels in various sports are characterized by an average or advanced biological maturity status. Whatever the criteria used or the competitive level observed, studies point to the same direction, with very few exceptions. One of these is ice hockey competitors who tend to be characterized by a slight developmental delay; Buckler and Brodie (1977) also noted a retardation in a sample of 99 gymnasts competing at an interscholastic level. These data diverge somewhat from the observations of Caldarone, Léglise, Giampietro, and Berlutti (1986). In contrast to males, female athletes are usually delayed in their biological maturity status (see Tables 1.9 and 1.10). Gymnasts, ballet dancers, and figure skaters are the most delayed, followed by divers, tennis players, and, thereafter, track-and-field athletes, rowers, and volleyball players. Canoeists, alpine skiers, basketball players, handball players, swimmers, and synchronized swimmers are average in their maturity status. Some evidence indicates that top level swimmers are even slightly advanced.

There is some indication that in boys, the most marked advancement in maturity status is observed in pubescence, which is most probably due to the size, physique, composition, and performance advantage of early-maturing boys at these age levels. This advantage vanishes as boys approach adulthood, in which period late-maturing boys catch up. Furthermore, some studies suggest that in team sports, there are differences in maturity status as a function of the position of the players on the field. More extensive data are need to further clarify this.

Most of the literature concerning maturity characteristics in female athletes concentrates on age at menarche (see Malina, 1983; Märker, 1981). Consequently, several hypotheses have been proposed to explain the delay of menarche in female competitors in most sports. Probably one of the most popular hypotheses is that *training* delays menarche (Frisch et al., 1981). According to Malina (1984b), "the data dealing with intensive training and menarche are quite limited, associational, speculative, and do not control for other factors which influence the time of menarche" (p. 70). The conclusions arrived at by Frisch et al. (1981) are based upon a correlational analysis that does not imply a cause-effect sequence. If there is an association between training and menarche, the suggested underlying explanatory mechanism is hormonal. Currently, data are lacking in which the cumulative effects of hormonal responses to regular training in premenarcheal girls have been studied. Furthermore, it has been suggested that a certain level of fatness, which in turn is influenced by vigorous exercise, is needed to attain menarche (Frisch et al., 1973). As already discussed, the data do not support the specificity of fatness as a critical variable for menarche. Also, the questions remain unanswered as to why there is a positive association in male athletes and a negative association in female athletes, given that the underlying hormonal mechanisms of biological maturation are essentially the same, and why elite female swimmers

Table 1.7 Maturity Criteria and Characteristics of Young Male Athletes in Team Sports

Sport	Competitive level	Age (years)	Criterion	Characteristics	Authors
Baseball	Little League	12.5	Pubic hair	17% pubescent 45.5% postpubescent	Hale (1956)
	Little League	11-14	Skeletal age	5% delayed (CA) 45% average (CA) 45% advanced (CA)	Krogman (1959)
	Little League and senior high school	9-18	Skeletal age	Average (NP)	Clarke (1971)
Football	Interscholastic	10-15	Skeletal age	Advanced (NP)	Clarke (1971)
	Local league	10-14	Pubic hair	Average (U.S. sample)	Malina (1988)
Basketball	Interscholastic	9-12	Skeletal age	Average (NP)	Clarke (1971)
	Interscholastic	13-15	Skeletal age	Advanced (NP)	Clarke (1971)
	Interscholastic	15-17	Skeletal age	Average (NP)	Clarke (1971)
Soccer	Provincial	11.3 ± 0.8	Skeletal age	Average (CA)	Vrijens & Van Cauter (1985)
Ice hockey	International tournament	10-13	Skeletal age	Slightly delayed (CA)	Bouchard, Roy, & Larue (1969)
	Brno	12-15	Skeletal age	Delayed (CA + NP)	Kotulán, Reznicková, & Placheta (1980)

Note. CA = chronological age used as reference, and NP = nonparticipant control group.

Table 1.8 Maturity Criteria and Characteristics of Young Male Athletes in Individual Sports

Sport	Competitive level	Age (years)	Criterion	Characteristics	Authors
Cycling	Brno	12-15	Skeletal age	Advanced (NP & CA)	Kotulán, Řezníčková, & Placheta (1980)
Gymnastics	Interscholastic	10-19	Pubic hair and genital development	Delayed (British sample)	Buckler & Brodie (1977)
	International tournament	15-18	Skeletal age	Advance (CA)	Caldarone et al. (1986)
Rowing	Brno	12-15	Skeletal age	Advanced (NP + CA)	Kotulán et al. (1980)
Swimming	National competition	10-15	Skeletal age	Advanced (CA)	Szabó (1969)
	National competition	8-15	Skeletal age	Advanced (CA)	Bugyi & Kausz (1970)
	National competition	10-12	Genital development	Average (CA)	Thompson et al. (1974)
	National competition	8-18	Pubic hair and genital development	Average (CA)	Kanitz & Bar-Or (1974)
	Age-group and national competition	16.7 ± 1.0	Skeletal age	Average (U.S. sample) "best" advanced	Meleski (1980)
	Olympic competition	10-17	Skeletal age	Advanced (CA)	Malina (1982)
	National competition	9-12	Skeletal age	Advanced	Beunen et al. (1981-1982)
Track and field	Interscholastic	12-15	Skeletal age	Average (NP)	Clarke (1971)
	Interscholastic	15-17	Skeletal age	Advanced (NP)	Clarke (1971)
	Interscholastic	15-16	Skeletal age	Average (NP)	Clarke (1971)
	National competition	17-18	Skeletal age	Advanced (CA)	Malina et al. (1986)
				Average to slightly delayed (CA)	

Note. CA = chronological age used as reference, and NP = nonparticipant control group.

Table 1.9 Maturity Criteria and Characteristics of Young Female Athletes in Individual Sports

Sport	Competitive level	Age (years)	Criterion	Characteristics	Authors
Gymnastics	Olympic aspirants	10-16	Skeletal age	Delayed (NP)	Novotný & Taftlová (1979)
	National competition	11-16	Skeletal age	Delayed (CA)	Beunen, Claessens, & Van Esser (1981)
	Talented national competition	8-14	Breast development and pubic hair	Delayed (NP)	Peltenburg et al. (1984)
	Nontalented	8-14	Breast development and pubic hair	Delayed (NP)	Peltenburg et al. (1984)
Swimming	Olympic competition	under 17	Skeletal age	Slightly advanced (CA)	Malina et al. (1982)
	National competition	8-15	Skeletal age	Slightly advanced (CA)	Bugyi & Kausz (1970)
	National competition	7-16	Skeletal age	Average (CA)	Thompson et al. (1974)
	National competition	10-12	Breast development and pubic hair	Slightly advanced (F-SF)	Bar-Or (1975)
	Age-group and national competition	8-18	Breast development and pubic hair	Average, "best" advanced	Meleski (1980)
	Olympic competition	Under 16	Skeletal age	Advanced (CA)	Malina (1982)
	National competition	10-17	Skeletal age	Slightly advanced (CA), best average to slightly advanced	Beunen et al. (1981-1982)
	National competition	7-14	Breast development and pubic hair	Average (NP)	Peltenburg et al. (1984)
Track and field	Rostock	11-12	Skeletal age	Delayed (CA)	Labitzke & Vogt (1971)
	National competition	15-17	Skeletal age	Delayed (CA)	Malina et al. (1986)

Note. CA = chronological age used as reference, NP = nonparticipant control group, and F-SF = finalists compared to semifinalists.

Table 1.10 Mean Age at Menarche in Athletes Grouped by Sport

Sports	Age at menarche (mean ± SD)
Individual	
Skiing	12.9 ± 0.9
Canoeing	13.0 ± 1.1
Swimming	13.1 ± 1.3; 13.1 ± 1.0; 12.9; 13.1 ± 1.2; 13.9
Rowing	13.7 ± 1.1
Track and field	13.4 ± 2.1; 14.3 ± 1.6; 13.1 ± 1.0; 13.5 ± 1.1; 13.6 ± 1.3; 13.6 ± 1.8; 13.2 ± 1.3; 13.8
Tennis	14.0 ± 1.4
Diving	14.0 ± 1.1
Figure skating	14.0 ± 1.3; 15.0 ± 1.1
Ballet	13.7 ± 1.2; 15.4 ± 1.9
Gymnastics	14.5 ± 0.8; 15.1 ± 1.7; 15.0 ± 1.1; 13.7 ± 0.9
Team	
Basketball	13.3 ± 1.0; 13.1 ± 1.0
Handball	13.0 ± 1.0; 13.3 ± 1.0
Synchronized swimming	13.0 ± 1.4; 12.5
Volleyball	13.1 ± 0.9; 13.7 ± 0.7; 14.2 ± 0.9; 12.7 ± 1.0

Note. The appropriate reference data for the populations from which the athletes originate range from 12.5-13.4 years of age. Data from "Menarche in Athletes: A Synthesis and Hypothesis" by R.M. Malina, 1983, *Annals of Human Biology, 10*(1), pp. 3-6. Copyright 1983. Adapted by permission.

are, on the average, slightly advanced in biological age, although they also start intensive training at an early age. There is an association between age at menarche and skeletal maturation, and from the few longitudinal studies on the relationship between training and skeletal age, there is no evidence that skeletal age is affected by regular physical training (Malina, 1984b). Finally, as shown by Märker (1981) on the basis of 242 elite female athletes, the age of first parturition is not significantly influenced by hard training.

Among the factors that could partly explain the associations between biological age and performance capacity, the two-part hypothesis formulated by Malina (1983) is appealing and takes into account the evidence gathered thus far. This hypothesis combines biological selective factors (i.e., physique and skill) and social factors. A first part of the hypothesis states that the physique characteristics associated with later maturation in girls are generally more suitable for successful athletic performance. Successful female athletes with the appropriate physique and skill are thus selected by self and/or by parents and coaches. The second part of the hypothesis relates to the socialization process. Early-maturing girls are socialized away from sports participation, whereas late-maturing girls are socialized into sports participation. Data on the socialization of young girls are not extensive, of which most of the information comes from studies on white, male, high school, and college athletes or top-level amateurs (Coackley, 1987). For boys, sports participation is seen as being directly linked to their development as men. In the case of girls, sports participation is seldom associated with becoming women. Perhaps, with changing attitudes towards physical activity and physical fitness and with the increased acceptance of women as athletes, this perception will change. This two-part hypothesis probably does not constitute a complete explanation, and it is highly likely that factors such as family size, sociocultural phenomena, diet, and body composition need to be considered more carefully.

CONCLUSION AND CHALLENGES FOR FUTURE RESEARCH

It can be concluded that, at present, biological maturity status is most commonly assessed on the basis of sexual, morphological, dental, or skeletal criteria. Skeletal age is considered as the best single maturational index and is most often estimated from the hand and wrist by means of the atlas technique (Greulich & Pyle, 1950, 1959) or the bone-specific approach (Tanner & Whitehouse, 1959; Tanner, Whitehouse, Cameron et al., 1983; Tanner, Whitehouse, & Healy, 1962; Tanner, Whitehouse, Marshall et al., 1975). At younger ages, the technique developed by Roche et al. (1975b) for the knee is the most appropriate one. Skeletal age, sexual development, and a number of morphological maturity criteria are interrelated, but it is not possible to predict one of these from the other criteria on an individual basis. Nevertheless, the relationships among the maturity criteria are strong enough to define the general maturity status of a group of children or a given population.

Early-maturing boys and girls are advanced in their physical growth at all ages. They also have a greater lean body mass, fat mass, and heart volume. Moreover, a slight, but consistent, association is found between body type and biological age. The data do not support the specificity of weight or fatness as a critical variable in the occurrence of the first menstruation. During prepubescence, static strength is positively related to biological maturity in both boys and girls. The associations with other gross motor performance components are only moderate and are partially explained by size difference of early- and late-maturing children. In adolescent girls, only static strength is positively related to biological age, whereas in boys from 14 years on, all motor abilities are positively associated with biological age. In adolescent boys, the interaction between skeletal age and chronological age as such or in association with height or weight explains the largest proportion of the variance in motor performance. The explained variance is, however, not high enough to be of any predictive value. Young female athletes tend to be characterized by delayed biological maturity status, especially in gymnastics, figure skating, and ballet, whereas young male athletes are average in their maturity status or tend to be advanced in several sports. Some evidence indicates that maturity status is related to the field position in team sports and that advanced maturity is most pronounced in prepubescent and pubescent boys.

Most of our knowledge on the maturity-performance associations is based upon correlational analyses that do not indicate any cause-effect sequences. It is plainly evident that, when skeletal age is associated with static strength, there must be an underlying mechanism that explains this link. There is thus a need for more detailed studies, in which the underlying mechanism of the associations discussed in this paper are investigated. Long-term experiments, if ethically acceptable, or long-term natural experiments, in which existing groups of children living under given circumstances (e.g., participation in an intensive training program in a specific sports discipline) would tell us more about these mechanisms. Multidisciplinary studies, in which biological, sociological, and psychological factors are considered, would provide the most complete information. In these studies, a large number of biological factors needs to be examined: biological maturity characteristics, hormonal secretions, anthropometric dimensions, body composition, body type, physical performance components, specific sports skills, daily physical activity, and training.

From this discussion, it is clear that biological maturity status should be considered in the evaluation of the performance capacities of growing children. The point is not that the performance capacity of a youngster can be predicted from maturity status, even in combination with chronological age and size (height and weight), but rather that chronological age, maturity, and size are confounded in their effects on performance, and this influence must be taken into account. In this respect, it can be argued that in youth sports, especially during adolescence, children should be classified into biological, instead of chronological, age groups. The assignment of children to homogeneous groups is certainly not a new concept (Espenschade, 1963). Age, sex, height, and weight have often been proposed as a basis for classification. According to the analyses of Beunen et al. (1981), the interaction between biological age, chronological age, and height or weight is the most appropriate basis of classification for adolescent boys. But this is certainly not very practical, which points up the need for a simple maturational index that could be easily determined and would be of theoretical value. Although skeletal age is the best single maturational index, it is certainly not easy to assess, and considerable training is needed before acceptable levels of accuracy in skeletal age assessment are reached.

Some authors (Mészáros, Mohacsi, Szabó, & Szmodis, 1985; Wutscherk, 1974) have proposed the use of anthropometric data to estimate biological age. However, these authors overlook a fundamental principle that applies to every biological maturity characteristic: Eventually, all subjects must reach the same adult value. This is probably not the case for the above-noted anthropometric dimensions or combinations of them. Conceptually, such predictions are thus unacceptable. Another more promising possibility is the use of percentage of adult stature as a maturity index. As discussed previously, however, skeletal age functions as a predictor variable of adult height in the three most commonly practiced techniques. Notwithstanding, Roche, Tyleshevski, and Rogers (1983) demonstrated that in boys aged 5 to 15 years and in girls aged 3 to 13 years, skeletal age can be replaced in the prediction equation by chronological age. They recommend that this noninvasive method be used when irradiation cannot be justified or when invasion of personal privacy, as in estimating stages of sexual development, is inappropriate. What is needed, then, is population-specific reference data for percentage of adult stature to compare the individual value with age- and sex-specific reference values. Before this technique is applied extensively, it must be cross-validated in further research. Another approach that needs more detailed investigation is the technique proposed by Bock (1984) for the estimation of final height by fitting a triple-logistic growth function to individual height data. In this technique, it is possible to use a single height measurement in combination with the established growth characteristics of height to predict adult height.

Closely related to the problem of assigning children to homogeneous groups is the question of whether it is appropriate to construct reference data with skeletal age or some other variable as a reference basis instead of chronological age. It has been shown that the characteristics of the individual growth process are spread along the time axis when analyzed as a function of chronological age. These could be better related to biological milestones such as age at peak height velocity (Tanner, 1962). However, cross-sectional reference data are only useful in answering the question concerning how big, strong, and fast a child is for a given age and sex. For practical reasons, it is thus recommended to use chronological age as the reference basis. Indeed, in most situations where an evaluation of the physical performance capacities is required, neither skeletal age, nor, in some instances, height or weight is readily available. From a theoretical viewpoint, reference data in which physical performance capacities are plotted against a combination of chronological age, skeletal age, height, or weight are to be preferred.

As a final conclusion, it should be stressed that biological maturity is an important biological process that is related to growth and physical performance. Sport scientists, pediatricians, sport medical doctors, physical educators, and coaches must be aware of these interrelations and take them into account in the evaluation of the physical performance capacity of youngsters.

REFERENCES

Acheson, R.M. (1954). A method of assessing maturity from radiographs. A report from the Oxford child health survey. *Journal of Anatomy,* **88**, 498-508.

Acheson, R.M. (1966). Maturation of the skeleton. In F. Falkner (Ed.), *Human development* (pp. 465-502). Philadelphia: Saunders.

Anderson, D.L., Thompson, G.W., & Popovich, F. (1975). Interrelationships of dental maturity, skeletal maturity, height and weight from age 4 to 14 years. *Growth,* **39**, 453-462.

Anderson, M., Hwang, S.C., & Green, W.T. (1965). Growth of the normal trunk in boys and girls during the second decade of life. *Journal of Bone and Joint Surgery,* **47**, 1554-1564.

Bar-Or, O. (1975). Predicting athletic performance. *The Physician and Sportsmedicine,* **3**, 81-85.

Barton, W.H., & Hunt, E.E., Jr. (1962). Somatotype and adolescence in boys: A longitudinal study. *Human Biology,* **34**, 254-270.

Bastos, F.V., & Hegg, R.V. (1986). The relationship of chronological age, body build, and sexual maturation to handgrip strength in schoolboys ages 10 through 17 years. In J.A.P. Day (Ed.), *Perspectives in kinanthropometry* (pp. 45-49). Champaign, IL: Human Kinetics.

Bayley, N. (1943a). Size and body build of adolescents in relation to rate of skeletal maturity. *Child Development,* **14**, 47-90.

Bayley, N. (1943b). Skeletal maturing in adolescence as basis for determining percentage of completed growth. *Child Development,* **14**, 1-46.

Bayley, N. (1946). Tables for predicting adult height from skeletal age and present height. *Journal of Pediatrics,* **28**, 49-64.

Bayley, N., & Pinneau, S.R. (1952). Tables for predicting adult height from skeletal age: Revised for use with Greulich-Pyle hand standards. *Journal of Pediatrics,* **40**, 423-441.

Beunen, G. (1973-1974). Somatotype and skeletal maturity in boys 12 through 14. *Hermes* (Leuven, English issue), **8**, 411-422.

Beunen, G., Claessens, A., Lefevre, J., Ostyn, M., Renson, R., & Simons, J. (1987). Somatotype as related to age at peak velocity and to peak velocity in height, weight, and static strength in boys. *Human Biology*, **59**, 641-655.

Beunen, G., Claessens, A., Ostyn, M., Renson, R., Simons, J., & Van Gerven, D. (1982). Skeletal maturation (TW2) and somatotype. In H. Lavallée & R.J. Shephard (Eds.), *Frontiers of activity and child health* (pp. 115-123). Québec: Editions du Pélican.

Beunen, G., Claessens, A., & Van Esser, M. (1981). Somatic and motor characteristics of female gymnasts. *Medicine and Sport*, **15**, 176-185.

Beunen, G., Malina, R.M., Ostyn, M., Renson, R., Simons, J., & Van Gerven, D. (1982). Fatness and skeletal maturity of Belgian boys 12 through 17 years of age. *American Journal of Physical Anthropology*, **59**, 387-392.

Beunen, G., Malina, R.M., Ostyn, M., Renson, R., Simons, J., & Van Gerven, D. (1983). Fatness, growth and motor fitness of Belgian boys 12 through 20 years of age. *Human Biology*, **55**, 599-613.

Beunen, G., Ostyn, M., Renson, R., Simons, J., Swalus, P., & Van Gerven, D. (1974). Skeletal maturation and physical fitness of 12 to 15 year old boys. *Acta Paediatrica Belgica*, **28**, 221-232.

Beunen, G., Ostyn, M., Renson, R., Simons, J., & Van Gerven, D. (1976). Skeletal maturation and physical fitness of girls aged 12 through 16. *Hermes* (Leuven, English issue), **10**, 445-457.

Beunen, G., Ostyn, M., Renson, R., Simons, J., & Van Gerven, D. (1979). Growth and maturity as related to motor ability. *South-African Journal for Research in Sport, Physical Education and Recreation*, **3**, 9-15

Beunen, G., Ostyn, M., Simons, J., Renson, R., & Van Gerven, D. (1981). Chronological and biological age as related to physical fitness in boys 12 to 19 years. *Annals of Human Biology*, **8**, 321-331.

Beunen, G., Ostyn, M., Simons, J., Van Gerven, D., Swalus, P., & De Beul, G. (1978). A correlational analysis of skeletal maturity, anthropometric measures and motor fitness of boys 12 through 16. In F. Landry & W.A.R. Orban (Eds.), *Biomechanics of sports and kinanthropometry* (pp. 343-349). Miami: Symposia Specialists.

Beunen, G., Simons, J., Ostyn, M., Renson, R., Van Gerven, D., Claessens, A., & Wellens, R. (1981-1982). Fysiek prestatievermogen en biologische maturiteit [Physical performance as related to biological maturation]. *Werken van de Belgische Vereniging voor Sportgeneeskunde en Sportwetenschappen*, **30**, 97-111.

Beunen, G., Wellens, R., Ostyn, M., Renson, R., Simons, J., Van Gerven, D., Claessens, A., Lefevre, J., & Van Reusel, B. (1988). *Skeletal maturation (TW2) as related to physical fitness*. Unpublished manuscript.

Bielicki, T., (1975). Interrelationships between various measures of maturation rate in girls during adolescence. *Studies in Physical Anthropology*, **1**, 51-64.

Bielicki, T., Koniarek, J., & Malina, R.M. (1984). Interrelationships among certain measures of growth and maturation rate in boys during adolescence. *Annals of Human Biology*, **11**, 201-210.

Bock, R.D. (1984). Predicting the adult stature of preadolescent children. In C. Suzanne (Ed.), *Genetic and environmental factors during the growth period* (pp. 3-19). New York: Plenum.

Bookstein, F.C. (1978). The measurement of biological shape and shape change. New York: Springer Verlag.

Borms, J., Hebbelinck, M., & Ross, W.D. (1973). Somatotype and skeletal maturity in twelve year old boys. In O. Bar-or (Ed.), *Pediatric work physiology: Proceedings of the Fourth International Symposium* (pp. 85-91). Netanya: The Wingate Institue for Physical Education and Sport.

Borms, J., Hebbelinck, M., & Van Gheluwe, B. (1977). Early and late maturity in Belgian boys, 6 to 13 years of age, and its relation to body type. In O. Eiben (Ed.), *Growth and development, physique* (pp. 399-406). Budapest: Akadémiai Kiado.

Bouchard, C., Leblanc, C., Malina, R.M., & Hollmann, W. (1978). Skeletal age and submaximal working capacity in boys. *Annals of Human Biology*, **5**, 75-78.

Bouchard, C., Malina, R.M., Hollmann, W., & Leblanc, C. (1976). Relationship between skeletal maturity and submaximal working capacity in boys 8 to 18 years. *Medicine and Science in Sports*, **8**, 186-190.

Bouchard, C., Roy, B., & Larue, M. (1969). L'âge osseux des jeunes participants du Tournoi International de Hockey Pee-Wee de Québec [Skeletal age of young ice-hockey players participating in an International Pee-Wee Tournament in Quebec]. *Mouvement*, **4**, 225-232.

Buckler, J.M.H., & Brodie, D.A. (1977). Growth and maturity characteristics of schoolboy gymnasts. *Annals of Human Biology*, **4**, 455-463.

Bugyi, B, & Kausz, I. (1970). Radiographic determination of skeletal age of the young swimmers. *Journal of Sports Medicine and Physical Fitness*, **10**, 269-270.

Caldarone, G., Léglise, M., Giampietro, M., & Berlutii, G. (1986). Anthropometric measurements, body composition, biological maturation and growth predictions in young male gymnasts of high competitive level. *Journal of Sports Medicine*, **26**, 406-415.

Carron, A.V., Aitken, E.J., & Bailey, D.A. (1977). The relationship of menarche to the growth and development of strength. In H. Lavallée & R.J. Shephard (Eds.), *Frontiers of activity and child health* (pp. 139-143). Québec: Editions du Pélican.

Carron, A.V., & Bailey, D.A. (1974). Strength development in boys from 10 through 16 years. *Monographs of the Society for Research in Child Development, 39*(4, Serial No. 157).

Cheek, D.B., Schultz, R.B., Parra, A., & Reba, R.C. (1970). Overgrowth of lean and adipose tissues in adolescent obesity. *Pediatric Research, 4,* 268-269.

Clarke, H.H. (1971). *Physical and motor tests in the Medford boy's growth study.* Englewood Cliffs, NJ: Prentice Hall.

Clarke, H.H., & Degutis, E.W. (1962). Comparison of skeletal age and various physical and motor factors with the pubescent development of 10, 13, and 16 year old boys. *Research Quarterly, 33,* 356-368.

Clarke, H.H., & Harrison, J.C.E. (1962). Differences in physical and motor traits between boys of advanced, normal, and retarded maturity. *Research Quarterly, 33,* 13-25.

Coackley, J.J. (1987). Children and the sport socialization process. In D. Gould & M.R. Weiss (Eds.), *Advances in pediatric sport sciences: Vol. 2. Behavioral issues* (pp. 43-60). Champaign, IL: Human Kinetics.

Comité pour le Développement du Sport. (1987). *Eurofit. Manuel pour les tests Eurofit d'aptitude physique* [Eurofit. Manual for the Eurofit physical fitness test battery]. Strasbourg: Conseil de l'Europe.

Crampton, C.W. (1908). Physiological age: A fundamental principle. *American Physical Education Review, 8,* 3-6.

Cumming, G.R. (1973). Correlation of athletic performance and aerobic power in 12 to 17 year old children with bone age, calf muscle, total body potassium, heart volume, and two indices of anaerobic power. In O. Bar-Or (Ed.), *Pediatric work physiology: Proceedings of the Fourth International Symposium* (pp. 109-134). Netanya: The Wingate Institute for Physical Education and Sport.

Damon, A., & Bajema, C.J. (1974). Age at menarche: Accuracy of recall after thirty nine years. *Human Biology, 46,* 381-384.

Damon, A., Damon, S.T., Reed, R.B., & Valadian, I. (1969). Age at menarche of mothers and daughters, with a note on accuracy of recall. *Human Biology, 41,* 161-175.

Demirjian, A. (1978). Dentition. In F. Falkner & J.M. Tanner (Eds.), *Human growth: 2. Postnatal growth* (pp. 413-444). New York: Plenum.

Demirjian, A., & Goldstein, H. (1976). New systems for dental maturity based on seven and four teeth. *Annals of Human Biology, 3,* 411-414.

Demirjian, A., Goldstein, H., & Tanner, J.M. (1973). A new system for dental age assessment. *Human Biology, 45,* 211-227.

Dupertuis, C.W., & Michael, N.B. (1953). Comparison of growth in height and weight between ectomorphic and mesomorphic boys. *Child Development, 24,* 203-214.

Ellis, J.D., Carron, A.V., & Bailey, D.A. (1975). Physical performance in boys from 10 through 16 years. *Human Biology, 47,* 263-281.

Ellison, P.T. (1981). Prediction of age at menarche from annual height increments. *American Journal of Physical Anthropology, 56,* 71-75.

Espenschade, A.S. (1940). Motor performance in adoloscence including the study of relationhips with measures of physical growth and maturity. *Monographs of the Society for Research in Child Development, 5*(1, Serial No. 24).

Espenschade, A.S. (1963). Restudy of the relationships between physical performances of school children and age, height and weight. *Research Quarterly, 34,* 144-153.

Falkner, F. (1958). Skeletal maturation: An appraisal of concept and method. *American Journal of Physical Anthropology, 16,* 381-396.

Falkner, F., & Tanner, J.M. (1978). Introduction. In F. Falkner & J.M. Tanner (Eds.), *Human growth: 1. Principles and prenatal growth* (pp. IX-X). New York: Plenum.

Finney, D.J. (1952). *Probit analysis.* Cambridge: University Press.

Frisch, R. (1974). A method of prediction of age of menarche from height and weight at ages 9 through 13 years. *Pediatrics, 53,* 384-390.

Frisch, R.E., Gotz-Wilberger, A.V., McArthur, J.W., Albright, T., Witschi, J., Bullen, B., Birnholz, J., Reed, R.B., & Hermann, H. (1981). Delayed menarche and amenorrhea of college athletes in relation to age of onset of training. *Journal of the American Medical Association, 246,* 1559-1563.

Frisch, R.E., & Revelle, R. (1970). Height and weight at menarche and a hypothesis of critical body weights and adolescents. Science, *169,* 397-399.

Frisch, R.E., Revelle, R., & Cook, S. (1973). Components of weight at menarche and the initiation of the adolescent growth spurt in girls: Estimated total water, lean body weight and fat. *Human Biology, 45,* 469-483.

Garn, S.M., Cheek, D.C., & Guire, K.E. (1975). Growth, body composition and development of obese and lean children. In M. Winick (Ed.), *Childhood obesity* (pp. 23-46). New York: Wiley.

Garn, S.M., Clark, D.C., & Guire, K.E. (1974). Level of fatness and size attainment. *American Journal of Physical Anthropology, 40,* 447-450.

Garn, S.M., & Haskell, J.A. (1959). Fat and growth during childhood. *Science, 130,* 1711-1712.

Garn, S.M., & Haskell, J.A. (1960). Fat thickness and developmental status in childhood and adolescence. *American Journal of Diseases in Childhood, 99,* 746-751.

Goldstein, H. (1984). Current developments in the design and analysis of growth studies. In J. Borms, R. Hauspie, A. Sand, C. Suzanne, & M. Hebbelinck (Eds.), *Human growth and development* (pp. 733-572). New York: Plenum.

Greulich, W.W., & Pyle, I. (1950). *Radiographic atlas of skeletal development of the hand and wrist*. Stanford: Stanford University Press.

Greulich, W.W., & Pyle, I. (1959). *Radiographic atlas of skeletal development of the hand and wrist* (2nd edition). Stanford: Stanford University Press.

Hale, J.C. (1956). Physiological maturity of Little League baseball players. *Research Quarterly, 27*, 276-284.

Hebbelinck, M., Borms, J., & Clarys, J. (1971). La variabilité de l'âge squelettique et les corrélations avec la capacité de travail chez des garçons de 5me année primaire [The variability in skeletal age and its correlation with working capacity in boys of the 5th grade]. *Kinanthropologie, 3*, 125-135.

Hebbelinck, M., Borms, J., Duquet, W., & Vanderwaeren, M. (1986). Relationships between skeletal age and physical fitness variables of 6-year-old children. In J.A.P. Day (Ed.), *Perspectives in kinanthropology* (pp. 51-56). Champaign, IL: Human Kinetics.

Hewitt, D., & Acheson, R.M. (1961). Some aspects of skeletal development through adolescence: 2. The inter-relationship between skeletal maturation and growth at puberty. *American Journal of Physical Anthropology, 19*, 333-344.

Hollmann, W., & Bouchard, C. (1970). Untersuchungen über die Beziehungen zwischen chronologischem und biologischem Alter zu spiroergometrischen Messgrössen, Herzvolumen, anthropometrischen Daten and Skelettmuskelkraft bei 8-18 jährigen Jungen [Relations between chronological, skeletal age and ergometric characteristics, heart volume, anthropometric dimensions and muscle strength in 8 to 18 year old boys]. *Zeitschrift für Kreislaufforschung, 59*, 160-176.

Hunt, E., Jr., Cocke, G., & Gallagher, J.R. (1958). Somatotye and sexual maturation in boys: A method of development analysis. *Human Biology, 30*, 73-91.

Johnston, F.E. (1964). The relationship of certain growth variables to chronological and skeletal age. *Human Biology, 36*, 16-27.

Johnston, F.E., & Malina, R.M. (1966). Age changes in the composition of the upper arm in Philadelphia children. *Human Biology, 38*, 1-21.

Jones, H.E. (1949). *Motor performance and growth. A developmental study of static dynamometric strength*. Berkeley: University of California Press.

Kanitz, M., & Bar-Or, O. (1974). Relationship between anthropometric, developmental and physiologic parameters and achievement in swimming in 10- to 12-year old boys (Abstract). *Israel Journal of Medical Sciences, 10*, 289.

Kelly, J., & Reynolds, L. (1947). Appearance and growth of ossification centres and increase in the body dimensions. *American Journal of Roentgenology*, **57**, 477-516.

Kemper, H.C.G., Verschuur, R., Ras, K.G.A., Snel, J., Splinter, P.G., & Tavecchio, L.W.C. (1975). Biological age and habitual physical activity in relation to physical fitness in 12- and 13-year old schoolboys. *Zeitschrift für Kinderheilkunde*, **119**, 169-179.

Koinzer, K. (1978). Zu den Unterschieden der ergometrischen Leistungsfähigkeit und der Sauerstoffaufnahmefähigkeit bei 10- bis 14 jährigen Kinderen und Jugendlichen in Abhängigkeit vom biologischen Entwicklungsstand [Differences in oxygen uptake and working capacity in 10 to 14 year old children classified according to their biological maturity status]. *Medizin und Sport*, **18**, 184-188.

Koinzer, K., Enderlein, G., & Herforth, G. (1981). Untersuchungen zur Abhängigkeit der W170 vom Kalenderalter, vom biologischen Entwicklungsstand und vom Übungszustand bei 10- bis 14-jährigen Jungen und Mädchen mittels dreifaktorieller Varianzanalyse [Association between PWC170, chronological age, skeletal age, and training status in 10 to 14 year old boys]. *Medizin und Sport*, **21**, 201-206.

Kotulán, J., Řezničková, M., & Placheta, Z. (1980). Exercise and growth. *Acta Facultatis Medicae Universitas Brunensis*, **67**, 61-118.

Krogman, W.A. (1959). Maturation age of 55 boys in Little League World Series 1957. *Research Quarterly*, **30**, 54-56.

Labitzke, H. (1971). Über Beziehungen zwischen biologischen Alter (Ossifikationsalter) und der Körperlänge, den Körpergewicht und der Körperoberfläche sowie der maximalen Sauerstoffaufnahme [Relationships between biological age (skeletal age), stature, weight, body surface, and oxygen uptake]. *Medizin und Sport*, **11**, 82-86.

Labitzke, H. & Vogt, M. (1971). Über den Einfluss eines ausdauerbetonten Trainings bei Mädchen unter den Bedingungen von Schulsportgemeinschaften [Influence of endurance training within school sport clubs for girls]. *Medizin und Sport*, **11**, 525-529.

Low, W.D., Chan, S.T., Chang, K.S.F., & Lee, M.M.C. (1968). Skeletal maturation of Southern Chinese children. *Child Development*, **35**, 1313-1366.

Malina, R.M. (1975). Anthropometric correlates of strength and motor performance. *Exercise and Sport Sciences Reviews*, **3**, 249-274.

Malina, R.M. (1978a). Adolescent growth and maturation: Selected aspects of current research. *Yearbook of Physical Anthropology*, **21**, 63-94.

Malina, R.M. (1978b). Growth of muscle tissue and muscle mass. In F. Falkner & J.M. Tanner (Eds.), *Human growth: Volume 2. Postnatal growth* (pp. 273-294). New York: Plenum.

Malina, R.M. (1978c). Physical growth and maturity characteristics of young athletes. In R.A. Magill, M.J. Ash, & F.L. Smoll (Eds.), *Children in sport: A contemporary anthology* (pp. 79-101). Champaign, IL: Human Kinetics.

Malina, R.M. (1982). Physical growth and maturity characteristics of young athletes. In R.A. Magill, M.J. Ash, & F.L. Smoll (Eds.), *Children in sport* (2nd ed., pp. 73-96). Champaign, IL: Human Kinetics.

Malina, R.M. (1983). Menarche in athletes: A synthesis and hypothesis. *Annals of Human Biology, 10*, 1-24.

Malina, R.M. (1984). Human growth, maturation, and regular physical activity. In R.A. Boileau (Ed.), *Advances in pediatric sport sciences: Vol. 1. Biological issues* (pp. 59-83). Champaign, IL: Human Kinetics.

Malina, R.M. (1986). Maturational considerations in elite young athletes. In J. Day (Ed.), *Perspectives in kinanthropometry* (pp. 29-43). Champaign, IL: Human Kinetics.

Malina, R.M. (1988). Biological maturity status of young athletes. In R.M. Malina (Ed.), *Young athletes: Biological, psychological and educational perspectives* (pp. 121-140). Champaign, IL: Human Kinetics.

Malina, R.M., Beunen, G., Wellens, R., & Claessens, A. (1986). Skeletal maturity and body size of teenage Belgian track and field athletes. *Annals of Human Biology, 13*, 331-339.

Malina, R.M., Bouchard, C., Shoup, R.F., Demirjian, A., & Larivière, G. (1982). Growth and maturity status of Montreal Olympic athletes less than 18 years of age. *Medicine and Sport, 16*, 117-127.

Malina, R.M., Meleski, B.W., & Shoup, R.F. (1982). Anthropometric, body compositions, and maturity characteristics of selected school-age athletes. *Pediatric Clinics of North America, 29*, 1305-1322.

Märker, K. (1981). Influence of athletic training on the maturity process of girls. *Medicine and Sport, 15*, 117-126.

Marshall, W.A. (1974). Interrelationships of skeletal maturation, sexual development and somatic growth in man. *Annals of Human Biology, 1*, 29-40.

Marshsall, W.A. (1978). Puberty. In F. Falkner & J.M. Tanner (Eds.), *Human Growth: 2. Postnatal growth* (pp. 141-181). New York: Plenum.

Marshall, W.A., & Tanner, J.M. (1969). Variation in the pattern of pubertal changes in girls. *Archives of Disease in Childhood, 44*, 291-303.

Marshall, W.A. & Tanner, J.M. (1970). Variation in the pattern of pubertal changes in boys. *Archives of Disease in Childhood, 45*, 13-23.

Meleski, B.W. (1980). *Growth, maturity, body composition, and selected familial characteristics of competitive swimmers 8 to 18 years of age.* Unpublished doctoral dissertation, University of Texas, Austin.

Mészáros, J., Mohacsi, J., Szabó, T., & Szmodis, I. (1985). Assessment of biological development by anthropometric variables. In R.A. Binkhorst, H.C.G. Kemper, & W.H.M. Saris (Eds.), *Children and exercise XI* (Vol. 15, pp. 341-345). Champaign, IL: Human Kinetics.

Milman, D.H. & Bakwin, H. (1950). Ossification of metacarpal metatarsal centres as a measure of maturation. *Journal of Pediatrics*, **36**, 617-620.

Neinstein, L.S. (1982). Adolescent self-assessment of sexual maturation. *Clinical Pediatrics*, **21**, 482-484.

Nicholson, A.B., & Hanley, C. (1953). Indices of physiological maturity: Derivation and interrelationships. *Child Development*, **24**, 3-38.

Novotný, V.V. & Taftlová, R. (1971). Biological age and sport fitness of young gymnast women. In V.V. Novotný (Ed.), *Anthropological Congress dedicated to Ales Hrdlička* (pp. 123-130). Prague: Academia

Pařízková, J. (1977). *Body fat and physical fitness*. The Hague: Martinus Nijhoff.

Pařízková, J., & Čermák, J. (1977). Relationships between height, total and lean body weight, heart volume and bone in adolescent boys. In H. Lavallée & R.J. Shephard (Eds.), *Frontiers of activity and child health* (pp. 124-130). Québec: Editions du Pélican.

Peltenburg, A.L., Erich, W.B.M., Berninck, M.J.E., Zonderland, M.L., & Huisveld, I.A. (1984). Biological maturation, body composition, and growth of female gymnasts and control group schoolgirls and girl swimmers, aged 8 to 14 years: A cross-sectional survey of 1064 girls. *International Journal of Sports Medicine*, **5**, 36-42.

Petrovcic, F., Medved, R., & Horvat, V. (1957). Fixation de l'âge physiologique des jeunes a l'aide de la radiographie du squelette [Determination of physiological age by means of an x-ray of the skeleton]. In M. Mihovilovic (Ed.), *Congrès d'étude de la Fig. Partisan de Yugoslavie* (pp. 181-187). Zagreb: Fédération pour l'Education Physique.

Pryor, J.W. (1905). Development of the bone of the hand as shown by X-ray method. *Bulletin State College (Kentucky)*, Series 2(5).

Quaade, F. (1955). *Obese children*. Copenhagen: Danish Science Press.

Rajic, M.K., Brisson, G.R., Shephard, R.J., Lavallée, H., Jéquier, J.C., Massé, R., Jéquier, S., Lussier, T., & Labarre, R. (1979). Maturité osseuse et performance physique [Skeletal age and physical performance]. *Canadian Journal of Applied Sport Sciences*, **4**, 223-225.

Rarick, G.L., & Oyster, N. (1964). Physical maturity, muscular strength, and motor performance of young school-age boys. *Research Quarterly*, **35**, 523-531.

Reynolds, E.L. (1946). Sexual maturation and the growth of fat, muscle and bone in girls. *Child Development*, **17**, 121-144.

Reynolds, E.L., & Asakawa, H. (1951). Skeletal development in infancy: Standards for clinical use. *American Journal of Roentgenology, Radium Therapy and Nuclear Medicine,* **65,** 403-409.

Reynolds, E.L., & Wines, J.V. (1948). Individual differences in physical changes associated with adolescence in girls. *American Journal of Diseases of Children,* **75,** 329-350.

Reynolds, E.L., & Wines, J.V. (1951). Physical changes associated with adolescence in boys. *American Journal of Diseases of Children,* **82,** 529-547.

Richey, H.G. (1937). The relation of accelerated, normal and retarded puberty to the height and weight of school children. *Monographs of the Society for Research in Child Development,* **2**(Serial No. 8).

Roche, A.F. (1978). Bone growth and maturation. In F. Falkner & J.M. Tanner (Eds.), *Human growth: 2. Postnatal growth* (pp. 317-355). New York: Plenum.

Roche, A.F. (1980). The measurement of skeletal maturation. In F.E. Johnston, A.F. Roche, & C. Suzanne (Eds.), *Human physical growth and maturation. Methodologies and factors* (pp. 61-82). New York: Plenum.

Roche, A.F. (1984). Adult stature prediction: A critical review. *Acta Medica Auxologica,* **16,** 5-28.

Roche, A.F. Tyleshevski, F., & Rogers, E. (1983). Non-invasive measurements of physical maturity in children. *Research Quarterly for Exercise and Sport,* **54,** 364-371.

Roche, A.F., Wainer, H., & Thissen, D. (1975a). Predicting adult stature for individuals. *Monographs in Pediatrics,* **3,** 1-114.

Roche, A.F., Wainer, H., & Thissen, D. (1975b). *Skeletal maturity: Knee joint as a biological indicator.* New York: Plenum.

Rotch, T.M. (1909). A study of the development of the bones in children by roentgen method, with the view of establishing a developmental index for the grading of and the protection of early life. *Transactions of the American Association of Physicians,* **24,** 603-630.

Savov, S.G., (1978). Physical fitness and skeletal maturity in girls and boys 11 years of age. In R.J. Shephard & H. Lavallée (Eds.), *Physical fitness assessment: Practice and application* (pp. 222-228). Springfield, IL: Charles C Thomas.

Sawtell, R.O. (1929). Ossification and growth of children one to eight years of age. *American Journal of Diseases of Children,* **37,** 61-87.

Seils, L.R.G. (1951). The relationship between measures of physical growth and gross motor performance of primary-grade school children. *Research Quarterly,* **22,** 244-260.

Seltzer, C.C., & Mayer, J. (1964). Body build and obesity. Who are the obese? *Journal of the American Medical Association,* **189,** 103-110.

Shephard, R.J., Lavallée, H., Rajic, K.M., Jéquier, J.C., Brisson, G., & Beaucage, C. (1978). Radiographic age in the interpretation of physiological and anthropological data. In J. Borms & M. Hebbelinck (Eds.), *Pediatric work physiology, medicine and sport* (Vol. 11, pp. 124-133). Basel: Karger.

Shuttleworth, F.K. (1937). Sexual maturation and the physical growth of girls age six to nineteen. *Monographs of the Society for Research in Child Development*, 2(Serial No. 5).

Simmons, K. (1944). The Brush Foundation study of child growth and development: 2. Physical growth and development. *Monographs of the Society for Research in Child Development*, **9**, 1-87.

Szabó, S. (1969). Die Bedeutung und die Auswirkung des biologischen Lebensalter auf die Wettkampfergebnisse der Sportler im Pubertätsalter [The meaning and influence of biological age on the results of athletes during pubescence]. *Schweizerische Zeitschriift der Sportmedizin*, **17**, 47-65.

Szabó, S., Doka, J., Apor, R., & Somogyvari, K. (1972). Die Beziehung zwischen Knockenlebensalter, funktionellen anthropometrischen Daten und der aeroben Kapazität [Relationships between skeletal age, functional anthropometric dimensions and aerobic capacity]. *Schweizerische Zeitschrift für Sportmedizin*, **20**, 109-115.

Szabó, T., & Mészáros, J. (1980). Relationships of bone age, physical development and athletic performance at the age of 11 to 12 years. *Anthropologiai Közlemények*, **24**, 263-267.

Tanner, J.M. (1962). *Growth at adolescence*. Oxford: Blackwell Scientific Publications.

Tanner, J.M. (1981). *A history of the study of human growth*. London: Cambridge University Press.

Tanner, J.M., & Whitehouse, R.H. (1959). *Standards for skeletal maturity: Part 1*. Paris: International Children's Centre.

Tanner, J.M., Whitehouse, R.H., Cameron, N., Marshall, W.A., Healy, M.J.R., & Goldstein, H. (1983). *Assessment of skeletal maturity and prediction of adult height (TW2 method)*. London: Academic Press.

Tanner, J.M., Whitehouse, R.H., & Healy, M.J.R. (1962). *A new system for estimating skeletal maturity from the hand and wrist, with standards derived from a study of 2600 healthy British children: Part 2. The scoring system*. Paris: International Children's Centre.

Tanner, J.M., Whitehouse, R.H., Marshall, W.A., Healy, M.J.R., & Goldstein, H. (1975). *Assessment of skeletal maturity and prediction of adult height (TW2 method)*. London: Academic Press.

Taranger, J., Bruning, B., Claesson, I., Karlberg, P., Landström, T., & Lindström, B. (1976). A new method for the assessment of skeletal maturity—

the Mat-method (mean appearance time of bone stages). *Acta Paediatrica Scandinavica*, (Suppl. 258), 109-120.

Thompson, G.G., Blanksby, B.A., & Doran, G. (1974). Maturity and performance in age group competitive swimmers. *Australian Journal of Physical Education,* **64**, 21-25.

Tiisala, R., Kantero, R.L., & Tamminen, T. (1971). A mixed longitudinal study on skeletal maturation in healthy Finnish children aged 5-10 years. *Human Biology,* **43**, 224-236.

Todd, J.W. (1937). *Atlas of skeletal maturation: Part 1. Hand.* London: Mosby.

Vrijens, J., & Van Cauter, C. (1985). Physical performance capacity and specific skills in young soccer players. In R.A. Binkhorst, H.C.G. Kemper, & W.H.M. Saris (Eds.), *Children and exercise XI* (Vol. 9, pp. 285-292). Champaign, IL: Human Kinetics.

Wolff, O.H. (1955). Obesity in children: A study of the birth weight, the height, and the onset of puberty. *Quarterly Journal of Medicine,* **24**, 109-123.

Wutscherk, H. (1974). Die Bestimmung des "biologischen" Alters [The assessment of biological age]. *Theorie und Praxis der Körperkultur,* **23**, 159-170.

2

Short-Term Muscle Power in Children and Adolescents

Anthony Sargeant
Vrije Universiteit and Universiteit van Amsterdam

In the study of the development of physical capabilities in children and adolescents, the vast majority of published investigations have concentrated on aerobic function, usually assessed in terms of maximal oxygen uptake ($\dot{V}O_2$max). This concentration of research effort has been a direct result of the development of a reliable and valid methodology for measurement using objective criteria. So much activity concentrated on this single aspect of physical function has resulted in its becoming almost a synonym for *physical fitness* or *physical work capacity*. It is clear, however, that $\dot{V}O_2$max measures only one aspect of a child's functional capability.

Indeed, it could be argued that short-term power output, produced in exercise lasting for a few seconds, may be a more telling index of functional capability than the maximal level of (aerobic) power that can be sustained for some minutes. Exercise of such intensity and duration that it elicits $\dot{V}O_2$max is relatively uncommon, even in the life of active children, compared with the need for short bursts of high-intensity exercise lasting for a few seconds (e.g., running for a bus or sprinting up stairs).

For the purposes of this review, *short-term power output* is defined as the maximum mechanical power that can be delivered during exercise of up to 60-s duration, that is, exercise for which the predominant source of energy is anaerobic, being derived from either high-energy phosphates (ATP and PC) or anaerobic glycolysis. This does not, of course, exclude a minority contribution from aerobic pathways. Furthermore, this operational definition is used in acknowledgment of the fact that these three energy supply mechanisms are not recruited in a mutually exclusive sequence; rather, there is a gradual shift in proportional contribution depending upon the intensity and duration of exercise. Figure 2.1 illustrates the effect of these overlapping energy supply mechanisms on the maximum external power that can be delivered by 13-year-old boys in exercises of different durations.

The muscular power delivered for physical activity of short-term duration results from many factors: These include proportionate contribution of energy pathways, efficiency of energy transformation, muscle architecture and size, and patterns of recruitment and coordination. Because of the highly invasive nature and the difficulty, if not impossibility, of estimating the interaction of

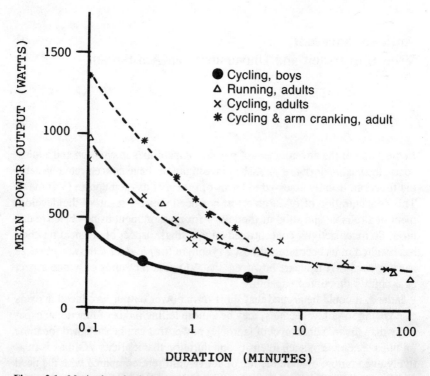

Figure 2.1 Maximal mechanical power (mean of one or more complete stroke cycles) delivered in exercise of different durations. Note semilogarithmic scale. *Note.* Children's data from Sargeant and Dolan, 1986; Adult data documented by Wilkie, 1960.

these various factors in the intact child, a number of tests have been developed that attempt to measure the external power delivered in a standardized test. This is not an unreasonable approach because it is indeed the resultant of these and other factors that defines the level of functional capability.

All of these tests have been developed on adults and subsequently, although infrequently and incompletely, applied to children and adolescents. The first section of this chapter discusses some of the tests that have been used in studies of children.

TESTS OF SHORT-TERM POWER

Fundamental Considerations

Short-term power output is predominantly dependent on energy supply intrinsic to the active muscle. Thus any test is very specific to the movement pattern used. We cannot expect information on the power output available in a movement involving leg muscles (e.g., cycling) to indicate anything about the functional status of the arm muscles. Neither can we assume that it will necessarily tell us anything about the short-term power output generated in another movement involving leg muscles, because the pattern of use and proportional contribution of the muscles involved may vary dramatically between the activities.

A major problem in attempting to assess maximal short-term power output is the dependence of power output upon the contraction velocity (Fenn & Marsh, 1935; Hill, 1922; Hill, 1938). Because the relationship between force and velocity is of an inverse curvilinear form, power, which is the product of these, has a parabolic relationship, with velocity reaching a maximum at some intermediate optimal velocity (Vopt); contraction at faster or slower velocities reduces power output (see Figure 2.2). As Wilkie (1960) pointed out, if a truly maximal power output is to be measured, it is important to closely match the external load to the capability of the active muscles so that they operate at their optimal velocity.

Methods

Vertical Jump Protocols. The measurement of maximal leg power by means of a vertical jump was first proposed by D.A. Sargent (1921) and L.W. Sargent (1924). Various modifications and increasingly sophisticated instrumentation have been developed over the years; however, the basic principle remains the same. Subjects are required to jump vertically as high as they can, and power is derived from either the height of the jump or the ground reaction forces and acceleration of the body center of mass (Davies & Rennie, 1968). It should be remembered that this test is measuring *instantaneous* power, probably

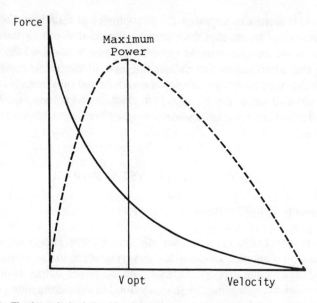

Figure 2.2   The theoretical relationship of muscle force to the velocity of contraction (solid line). Power is the mathematical product of force and velocity (dashed line).

reflecting the ability to transform ATP splitting into external power (Davies, Wemyss-Holden, & Young, 1984; Davies & Young, 1984; Ferretti, Gussoni, di Prampero, & Cerretelli, 1987). It is vital that the test be carefully standardized because profoundly different results can be obtained (e.g., by jumping with or without a counter movement; see Asmussen & Bonde-Petersen, 1974).

Many investigators tacitly assume that there is a natural matching of external load (the body weight) to the capability of the muscles to generate force and power, but few investigators have systematically examined this, either in adults or in children.

One recent report, based on experiments in which 12-year-old children performed jumps with added weight (from 5% to 30% body weight), indicated a linear decrease in peak power proportional to the added weight (Davies & Young, 1984). Thus it would seem that body weight is not less than the optimal load for maximal power output. This does not of course exclude the possibility that it could be more. Indeed, this is suggested by the fact that the inverse linear relationship shows no sign of a plateau around body weight. A further decrease of the external load (i.e., body weight) of 15% might be predicted to increase power output by about 80%. This could explain the difference that Davies and Young report between peak power in jumping and peak power in isokinetic cycling in these children (711 and 1,283 watts, respectively).

It is perhaps not surprising that the power of the leg muscles should lag behind the increase in the body weight during growth. It would be more surprising if the development of leg muscle power somehow anticipated the increase in body weight, which, as the natural external load, might be considered the stimulus for muscle development. However, a note of qualification should be added. Performance in vertical jumping is critically dependent upon the pattern of coordination of the active muscles. This may be especially significant for the action of the biarticular muscles, which transport useful power to distal joints (Bobbert, Hoek, van Ingen Schenau, Sargeant, & Schreurs, 1987). The change of external load may mean that the existing recruitment pattern is no longer optimal for maximal power production. Also, it is likely, at least in younger children, that the very complex and precise recruitment pattern required for maximal performance is not yet firmly established.

Running Tests. If, rather than instantaneous power, the investigator wants to estimate the power available in exercise where ATP resynthesis is necessary, then a more continuous form of exercise is required. Perhaps the most obvious of these is running. Hill (1970) illustrated such an experiment carried out by, and on, Charles Best in 1934, and Hill himself performed similar experiments before the Second World War (see also Elftman, 1940; Fenn, 1930). However, there is considerable difficulty in calculating the power generated in running on the flat. Furthermore, in a freely accelerating and, with fatigue, decelerating sprint, the relationship of power to velocity is not known. Margaria, Aghemo, and Rovelli (1966) proposed a simple but effective answer to these problems by asking subjects to run up a flight of stairs two steps at a time. By timing the speed and knowing the height ascended and body weight, they calculated the external power output generated in the first few seconds before fatigue occurred. The only equipment required was a timing device (e.g., photoelectric cells) and a suitable flight of stairs. Variability of this test was reported to be $\pm 4\%$. It should be noted that, although Margaria et al. (1966) first suggested a test protocol based on stair climbing, other investigators had previously used stair climbing to estimate human power output (e.g., Blix, 1906; Unna, 1946). However, the first real population data including measurements on children were presented by Margaria's group (see di Prampero & Cerretelli, Margaria, et al., 1966; Steplock, Veicsteinas, & Mariani, 1971).

Apart from simplifying the calculation of external power output, stair climbing also loads the active muscles with the subject's own body weight, and, as with jumping, it might be thought that functional development would be related to the normally imposed load—at least in a healthy, active population. However, some investigators have suggested that additional loading of adult subjects results in better optimization of the external load to muscle function (Caiozzo & Kyle, 1980; Kitagawa, Suzuki, & Miyashita, 1980). It is not known whether this observation also holds for children, or even whether it applies to all groups of adults. This contrasts with the Davies and Young (1984) study on the effects of external loading in jumping.

A number of investigators have collected data on children performing the stair-climbing test (Davies, Barnes, & Godfrey, 1972; di Prampero &

Cerretelli, 1969; Margaria et al., 1966; Steplock et al., 1971). In all of these studies there was an increase in maximal short-term power output expressed per kilogram of body weight between the ages of 10 and 20 years; however, after 20 to 30 years of age there is a rather similar decline in all groups except the highly self-selected group of Africans studied by di Prampero and Cerretelli (1969). Possible reasons for these age-related changes are discussed later in this chapter.

Cycle Ergometer Tests.   Alternatives to running tests are those based on cycling on stationary ergometers. Sprint tests based on cycling against known, constant braking forces have been used for many years (e.g., Benedict & Cathcart, 1913; Nielsen & Hansen, 1937; Nonweiler, 1958; Tuttle, 1949). Asmussen and Bøje (1945) used such a test in their classic paper on the effect of temperature on short-term power output. More recently, a number of groups have proposed protocols based on maximum effort performed against a fixed braking force (Ayalon, Inbar, & Bar-Or, 1974; Bar-Or, 1987; Crielaard & Pirnay, 1981; Cumming, 1973; Dotan & Bar-Or, 1983; Inbar & Bar-Or, 1986; Katch, Weltman, Martin, & Gray, 1977; Marechal, Pirnay, Crielaard, & Petit, 1979; Vandewalle, Peres, Heller, & Monod, 1985; Vandewalle, Peres, Heller, Panel, & Monod, 1987).

In test protocols where a single exercise bout is performed, it is important to set a braking force that matches the muscle's capability. In this way, true maximal power output can be measured at, or close to, optimal velocity. A number of authors have addressed the possibility of predicting the optimal braking force from body weight, but this issue has not been finally resolved, especially in the case of children (for review and discussion see Bar-Or, 1987). The use of body weight as the predictive index is not unreasonable because this is the external load normally imposed upon the muscle (e.g., during jumping and stair-climbing tests). However, there are two qualifications of which investigators must be aware.

First, during growth, but also as a consequence of illness, obesity, training, or disability, the normal relationship between body weight and leg muscle function may be variably dislocated. This makes it difficult, if not impossible, to predict the ideal braking force.

Second, an ideal braking force at the beginning of maximal exercise will not be ideal at the end of a test. Fatigue decreases the pedaling rate and thus power output is reduced as a consequence of a move away from the optimal pedaling rate for maximal power. This is simply the consequence of the power/velocity relationship in muscle (see Figure 2.2). The result is a reduction in power that is separate from, and additional to, that caused by fatigue. In 13-year-old boys, for example, the effect of pedaling at 60 $\text{rev} \cdot \text{min}^{-1}$ rather than at optimum (~ 120 $\text{rev} \cdot \text{min}^{-1}$) is to reduce maximal power by about 40% (Figure 2.3).

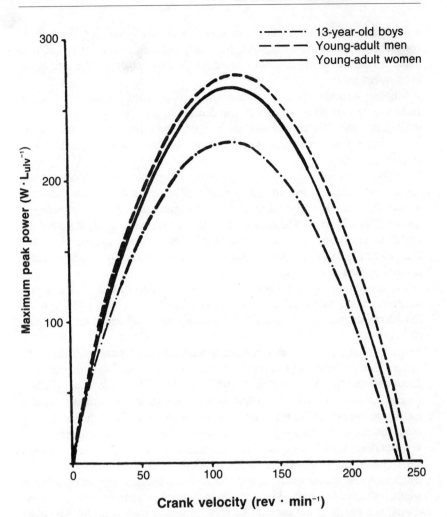

Figure 2.3 The relationship between the calculated maximum peak power and crank velocity during isokinetic cycling. Power is expressed in watts (W) and normalized for the anthropometrically determined muscle (plus bone) volume of the upper leg (L_{ulv}; see Figure 2.4). *Note.* From "Optimal Velocity of Muscle Contraction for Short-Term (Anaerobic) Power Output in Children and Adults" by A.J. Sargeant and P. Dolan. In *Children and Exercise XII* (p. 40) by J. Rutenfranz, R. Mocellin, and F. Klimt (Eds.), 1986, Champaign, IL: Human Kinetics. Copyright 1986 by Human Kinetics. Reprinted by permission.

In cognizance of these problems some authors have proposed the use of a series of very short tests (5-s duration) at different braking forces. In this way the optimum can be clearly identified and fatigue is not a problem (Marechal et al., 1979; Pirnay & Crielaard, 1979; Vandewalle et al. 1985; Vandewalle et al. 1987; Vandewalle, Peres, & Monod, 1984). This may be preferable to a single test in which a predicted ideal load is set. However, it is more time-consuming than a single test bout, especially because care must be taken to avoid a cumulative effect from muscle temperature changes and fatigue on subsequent bouts.

Whether a single test or a series is used, all tests are performed against a fixed load and involve acceleration and deceleration of the ergometer flywheel during the test. These changes are not usually taken into account when estimating the power output, but they can materially affect the calculation (Lakomy, 1986).

Sargeant, Hoinville, and Young (1981) developed an isokinetic cycle ergometer to control pedaling rate throughout an exercise test. The cranks of a cycle ergometer are driven through a variable speed gearbox by a large electric motor. The subjects, pedaling with the motor, attempt to speed it up but are unable to do so due to the characteristics of the motor's gear system. Nevertheless, effective force and power generated are monitored by means of strain gauges bonded to the cranks.

The derivation of force-velocity relationships using isokinetic ergometers suggests an optimal pedaling rate for maximal power of 110 to 120 rev•min^{-1} in both children and adults (Figure 2.3; McCarteney, Heigenhauser, Sargeant, & Jones, 1983; Sargeant & Dolan, 1986; Sargeant, Dolan, & Thorne, 1984; Sargeant et al., 1981). This optimal pedaling rate is probably influenced by factors such as the intrinsic character of the muscle, as expressed by fiber type, and muscle temperature (Sargeant, 1987; Sargeant, Dolan, & Young, 1984). Figure 2.3 also indicates that (a) there is no difference in the extrapolated value for maximum or optimum velocity between adults and children, (b) there is no difference in power output between young women and young men when it is standardized for the size of the active muscle, and (c) children's power output was significantly less than that of adults when standardized ($p < .01$). One might also suppose that the use of a standard crank length for all subjects would influence the optimal velocity, especially when comparing children and adults, but this does not seem to be very critical in studies of older children (Inbar, Dotan, Trousil, & Dvir 1983; Sargeant & Dolan, 1986).

One advantage of cycling tests is that they lend themselves to adaptation for the measurement of arm power. Care must be taken, however, to insure that the upper body is adequately restrained in these instances (see Davies & Sargeant, 1974). At present, few data are available on short-term power output of the arms in children (Blimkie, Roache, Hay, & Bar-Or, 1988; Inbar & Bar-Or, 1986).

Monoarticular Tests of Power. Human muscle power has been measured with ergometers that allow movement across a single joint (e.g., Bouisset, Cnockaert, & Pertuzon, 1966; de Koning, Binkhorst, Vos, & Van't Hof, 1985; Dern, Levene, & Blair, 1947; Hill, 1922; Ralston, Polissar, Inman, Close, & Feinstein, 1949; Wilkie, 1950). Recently, ergometers that control velocity of movement (isokinetic) have been made commercially available and enthusiastically promoted by their manufacturers. However, some particular problems exist in their application in research, as distinct from therapy. (See Bassey, Dudley, & Pearson, 1985; Perrine & Edgerton, 1978; Thomas, White, Sagar, & Davies, 1987; Vandewalle, Peres, & Monod, 1987; Wickiewicz, Roy, Powell, Perrine, & Edgerton, 1984; Winter, Wells, & Orr, 1981.) One problem is that it is difficult to voluntarily accelerate a limb segment up to optimal velocity for maximal power output in an isolated extension or flexion movement (see Sargeant et al., 1981, for a discussion of this point).

Despite these limitations some interesting work has been done using this approach, and it has clear value in measuring dynamic function of a group of muscles acting across one joint. (e.g., Thorstensson, Grimby, & Karlsson, 1976). Surprisingly few data are available for children.

NORMALIZATION OF DATA

Measurements of maximal power output are often expressed relative to the child's body weight. This may be a useful and appropriate standardization to make in assessing the child's functional capability for activity that requires the movement of body weight. Many daily activities are of this type, but in other activities (e.g., swimming, cycling, rowing, canoeing) there is not a direct link, and here such standardization is not so meaningful. Furthermore, it makes little sense to standardize arm muscle power for body weight. If one is interested in the intrinsic quality of the muscles being exercised it is important to have a measurement reflecting the dimensions of the active muscles. This approach has already been applied in relation to aerobic power in children and young adults and the measurement of muscle function in children (Davies, 1985; Davies & Sargeant, 1975; Davies et al., 1972). It seems logical to apply the same considerations to the measurement of short-term power output (Sargeant & Dolan, 1986).

This presents the investigator with a difficult problem. In complex multiarticular coordinated exercise such as running, jumping, cycling, or arm cranking, it is impossible to assess accurately the relative contribution of the active muscles. Even in monoarticular exercise such as knee extension the proportional contribution to power output from the active muscles is impossible to accurately assess. This would require detailed information on the length-tension and force-velocity condition prevailing in each of the contributing muscles during the power-producing movement. Accurate information of this kind is simply unobtainable in the intact human. Nevertheless, these difficulties should not be taken as a recipe for doing nothing. A number of informative and useful approaches are available for assessing muscle size.

Because the power produced by muscle is the resultant of all the sarcomeres in series and parallel, an estimate of the volume of the active muscle mass

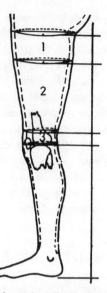

Figure 2.4 Schematic diagram of the leg to show division of the upper leg into a series of truncated cones to enable volume to be calculated according to the method of Jones and Pearson (1969). The dashed line indicates the boundary of the muscle plus bone cone. *Note.* From "Anthropometric Determination of Leg Fat and Muscle Plus Bone Volumes in Young Male and Female Adults" by P.R.M. Jones and J. Pearson, 1969, *Journal of Physiology, 204*, pp. 63-66P. Copyright 1969 by P.R.M. Jones and the *Journal of Physiology.* Adapted by permission.

Table 2.1 Linear Regression Equations Relating Four Uncompressed Roentgenogrammetic Values (*y*) to Equivalent Harpenden Skinfold Caliper Measurements (*x*) in mm for Children 6 to 15 Years Old.

Skinfold site	Sex	Regression	Correlation coefficient
Anterior thigh	M	$y = 0.39 + 0.59x$	.96
	F	$y = 0.27 + 0.50x$	.98
Posterior thigh	M	$y = 0.28 + 0.54x$	.98
	F	$y = 0.08 + 0.53x$	.98
Medial calf	M	$y = 0.48 + 0.51x$	.85
	F	$y = 0.57 + 0.51x$	.94
Lateral calf	M	$y = 1.12 + 0.43x$	.82
	F	$y = 1.77 + 0.38x$	.83

Note. Data from Jones, 1970.

may be the most useful measurement to make. In normal healthy children, for whom the use of X ray is unacceptable, the simplest technique is anthropometry. The limb is divided into segments that are treated as truncated cones (Figure 2.4). The volume of these is calculated by knowing the height and the diameters of the circular faces (Jones & Pearson, 1969). By measuring the thickness of the skin and subcutaneous fat layer, the researcher can calculate the cone volumes for the muscle-plus-bone core of the limb. This thickness can be estimated in children from measurements of skin folds made with Harpenden skin fold calipers using the regression equations given in Table 2.1 (Jones, 1970). With practice this measurement of limb and muscle-plus-bone volumes can be completed within 3 or 4 min. The accuracy in children of the measurement of total leg volume has been confirmed by comparison with volume determined from water displacement. If the heights of the anatomical landmarks defining the segments are carefully identified in an initial measurement and used thereafter, the repeatability is very high ($\pm 2\%$; Davies et al., 1972). The method can be applied to arms as well as legs (Sargeant & Davies, 1977a). It is possible with this technique to correct for the subcutaneous fat using skin fold thickness measured with calipers. The contribution of bone to the muscle-plus-bone volume is less easy to correct for, and there are no data for children; however, in *normal* adults bone constitutes a rather small and constant proportion of that volume ($11\% \pm 1\%$; cf. Sargeant & Davies, 1977b). It might be expected that a constant proportionality also exists in healthy children, even if different in magnitude. If so, it seems reasonable *not* to make an arbitrary correction but to express the volume as *muscle plus bone.*

The more serious difficulty with anthropometry is that it cannot distinguish between agonist and antagonist muscle in a limb segment. This presents a problem is some specific cases such as when a limb has been immobilized in a plaster cast, or in diseases that involve muscle atrophy of either primary or secondary origin. (Sargeant, Davies, Edwards, Maunder, & Young, 1977). Under normal circumstances there is likely to be some homogeneity of development within the muscles of a limb segment. In the future the application of nuclear magnetic resonance (NMR) imaging and grey scale ultrasound may become more widely available and enable a more precise measurement of muscle development in children without the hazard of ionizing radiation (Narici, Roi, & Landoni, 1988). In the meantime, at least anthropometric measurements of leg muscle plus bone volume should be made and reported.

FACTORS INFLUENCING MEASUREMENT

Muscle Temperature and Prior Exercise

One issue to carefully consider in testing human muscle function is the likely effect of variations in the temperature of the active muscles. Asmussen and

Bøje (1945) demonstrated a profound effect of increasing muscle temperature on the power output generated in an approximately 14-s maximal sprint on a cycle ergometer. Recently, the effect of changing muscle temperature on short-term maximum power at different contraction velocities (pedaling rate) has been described in a study by Sargeant (1987). These results are depicted in Figure 2.5. It should be noted that not only is maximum power increased by about 5% per °C rise in *muscle* temperature, but also that the optimum velocity for maximum power increases. In this study, optimum velocity for maximum power increased from 85 rev•min⁻¹ in the coldest conditions to 125 rev•min⁻¹ in the warmest.

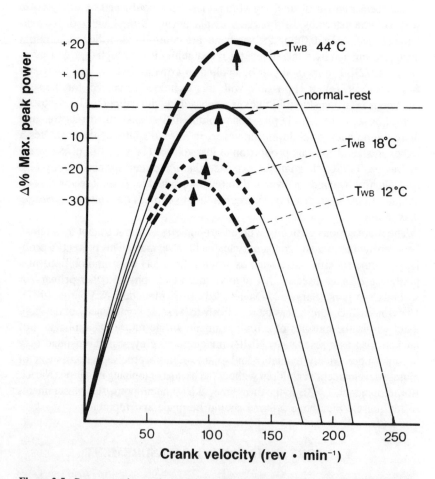

Figure 2.5 Percentage changes in maximum peak power in relation to velocity of contraction (pedaling rate) under four temperature conditions: after resting at normal room temperature of 21 °C and after 45 min of leg immersion in stirred water baths of different temperatures (T_{WB})—44, 18, and 12 °C. Quadriceps muscle temperature at 3 cm depth was 36.6, 39.3, 31.9, and 29.0 °C respectively in the four conditions. *Note.* Data from Sargeant, 1987.

Temperature changes in muscles can be brought about by both exercise and changes in the ambient temperature. With respect to the latter, limb muscles show a marked temperature gradient in cold weather with the more superficial layers falling by 5 or 6 °C compared with the deeper muscle. Children have a relatively large limb surface area to volume and thus may be especially vulnerable in this respect. Even at a normal room temperature of 21 °C, there is a significant temperature gradient of > 2 °C across adult leg muscles (Sargeant, 1987). This gradient may be steeper in children, but in both children and adults it is influenced by the thickness of the subcutaneous fat layer in the individual case. Due to the physiological mechanisms controlling body temperature, a somewhat higher than normal ambient air temperature may have a less critical effect upon muscle temperature and hence power output. In a study of 10- to 12-year-old children exposed to hot/dry or warm/humid environments, no systematic effect on power output could be detected (Dotan & Bar-Or, 1980). Unfortunately, Dotan and Bar-Or did not take measurements of muscle temperature. Furthermore, the data from heat exposure sessions with and without exercise-based warm-up were pooled, and this could have obscured any small effect.

The other major factor moderating muscle temperature is the immediate history of exercise, which presents the investigator with serious problems. Conventionally it has been common practice to allow subjects to warm-up by means of exercise before testing; however, unless carefully and rigorously standardized; this procedure can have significant and unpredictable consequences. A number of authors have measured the effect of exercise on muscle temperature in adults, and sometimes this has been related to short-term power output (e.g., Asmussen & Bøje, 1945; Bergh & Ekblom, 1979; Davies & Young, 1983; Sargeant, 1987). No equivalent data are available for children. Inbar and Bar-Or (1975) demonstrated an increase in power output following an intermittent, exercise-based warm-up in young boys but were unable to measure muscle temperature.

The possibility of a cumulative temperature effect from earlier exercise tests performed in the same session must be taken into account. This presents particular problems when a battery of tests are used. In addition to its effect upon muscle temperature, prior exercise may itself reduce the muscle power output in the short term due to fatigue (Ferretti et al., 1987; Margaria, di Prampero, Aghemo, Derevenco, & Mariani, 1971; Sargeant & Dolan 1987a) or in the long term as a consequence of persisting fatigue or actual damage (Friden, 1983; Jones, Newham, Round, & Tolfree, 1986; Sargeant & Dolan, 1987b). Alternatively, depending upon intensity and duration, prior exercise may elevate maximal short-term power output (Sargeant & Dolan, 1987a). This effect could be the result of an enhanced energy flux (Ferretti et al., 1987; Newsholme, 1978; Sahlin, 1986). Although none of these effects has been investigated in children, it is clear that prolonged strenuous exercise should be avoided in the days preceding a test of short-term power output. In addition, careful attention must be paid to the possible influence of any exercise undertaken immediately prior to the test, whether in the form of warm-up or as part of a larger battery of tests.

It may be the ideal to measure power output with the muscles at a homogenous and known temperature and in a stable metabolic state (i.e., from rest). However, given the difficulty and acceptability of deep muscle temperature measurements, especially in young children, it seems more pragmatic to take measurements under carefully standardized, normal conditions (e.g., after arriving at the laboratory, resting in a track suit at a room temperature of 21 °C). If a warm-up is considered desirable then it, too, should be standardized. These qualifications have particular relevance for longitudinal studies. A 1 °C difference in the mean muscle temperature at rest might easily be produced by seasonal variation in outside temperature or changes in clothing at the beginning compared to the end of a study. At optimal velocity for power production this might systematically change peak power output by 5%! It should be emphasized in this context that the effect of temperature is velocity dependent; thus, in a measurement of power output at a velocity greater than optimum, increases of 10% to 15% per °C are possible (Figure 2.5).

Age

A number of investigators have reported that short-term power output in children, even when standardized for body size, is consistently lower than that in young adults (e.g., Davies & Young, 1984; di Prampero & Cerretelli, 1969; Inbar & Bar-Or, 1986; Margaria et al., 1966; Sargeant, Dolan, & Thorne, 1985; Steplock et al., 1971). Even if standardization is made for the active muscle mass, a significant difference persists: Thirteen-year-old boys were 17% less powerful than either adult males or adult females when power was standardized for an anthropometric estimate of leg muscle plus bone volume (Sargeant & Dolan, 1986). Davies (1985) pointed out that some of the differences in muscle function between children and adults could be accounted for by rather small architectural changes in the muscle (e.g., in angle of pennation of fibers), but it remains to be investigated whether the differences in short-term power output could be accounted for by similar factors associated with, and determined by, the continuing growth in limb length during childhood.

Another possibility is that the young muscle is intrinsically less powerful in short-term exercise due to a restriction in the rate of resynthesis of ATP. However, because there is little evidence to suggest large differences in the resting levels of ATP and CP; *instantaneous* power could hardly be affected by this. Mean power would also be unaffected for some seconds until the level of high energy phosphate was depleted. Nevertheless, short-term power output *is* lower in children when measured in the first few seconds. It has been suggested that the maximal rate of anaerobic glycolysis may be lower in children than in adults, but this does not account for the child/adult differences observed in exercise of a few seconds' duration, although it could play a progressively important role in mean power output determined in tests lasting for more than 5 s.

The suggestion of a lower, age-dependent glycolytic rate is based on three observations. The first is that blood lactate concentration in children is not as high after intense exercise as it is in adults (e.g., Åstrand, 1952; Davies et al., 1972; Robinson, 1938). However, the interpretation of blood lactate concentration is fraught with difficulties because it is the resultant of not only lactate production via anaerobic glycolysis by the muscle cell, but also its rate of release into the circulation, its distribution in total body water, and its removal and breakdown by other tissues. Furthermore, this observation has recently been challenged by Cumming, Hastman, McCort, and McCullough (1980), who suggest that the difference may be illusory and largely a function of the duration of the final level sustained during $\dot{V}O^2max$ testing (under which condition the observation has most often been made). They report levels of blood lactate following routine maximal exercise testing in children that are comparable to adult values.

The second observation is that *muscle* lactate concentration measured from biopsy of the quadriceps during cycling exercise is lower in boys than in men at comparable levels of aerobic energy demand (Eriksson, 1972). This indicates lower steady state concentrations of muscle lactate at each exercise intensity; however, taken by itself, this still does not mean that the *maximum* rate at which anaerobic glycolysis could occur was necessarily lower in the boys than it was in the men.

Third, a more informative indicator of the maximal potential rate of glycolysis might be the activity of the controlling muscle enzymes. It has been suggested that phosphofructokinase (PFK) is an important rate-limiting enzyme for glycolysis. If so, then it may be pertinent that lower levels of PFK activity have been reported in muscle biopsies from the boys in the Ericksson (1972) study than in biopsies from men. However, some caution is necessary in assessing this evidence; enzyme activity is measured in vitro under optimal conditions, and this is certainly not the same as in vivo. Furthermore, it is worth noting that training increased PFK activity in the boys studied by Ericksson by almost 100%, but there is little to suggest that training increases anaerobic power independently of muscle size in this proportion (Rotstein, Dotan, Bar-Or, & Tenenbaum, 1986; Sargeant et al., 1985).

No unequivocal evidence confirms an age-dependent difference in the potential maximal rate of anaerobic glycolysis between children and adults. In any case, it is interesting to note that in electrical stimulation studies the muscle function of children, including an index of fatigue, is not different from that of adults if some dimensional corrections are made (Davies, 1985; Davies, White, & Young, 1983). Also, decreases in short-term power output after 20-30 years of age are of similar magnitude but the reverse of those seen during growth in children (Figure 2.6).

Apart from dimensional changes associated with growth, other factors could contribute to the increase in power output with age in children. These include

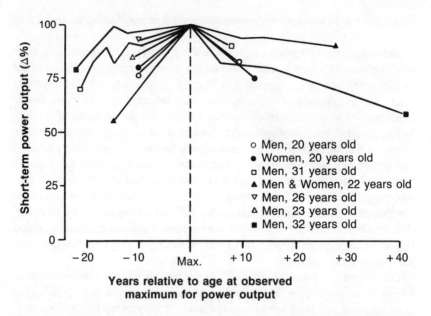

Figure 2.6　Selected maximum short-term (peak) power output data standardized for body weight. The cross-sectional data derived from the literature are plotted as a percentage change from the age at which the highest value was reported. This age is given for each reference. *Note.* Data from Davies, 1971; Davies, Barnes, and Godfrey, 1972; Davies and Young, 1984; Inbar and Bar-Or, 1986; Margaria, Aghemo, and Rovelli, 1966; Sargeant and Dolan, 1986; and Steplock, Veicsteinas, and Mariani, 1971.

changes in the density of myofibrillar packing in the muscle fibers, more effective transmission of power via connective tissue changes, better neural organization and activation, and changes in mean contractile speed of the muscle.

Learning and Motivation

No objective criteria exist that enable the investigator to confirm whether a truly maximal effort has been made in the sort of tests here described. Hence, the investigator is absolutely dependent on the willing cooperation of subjects being tested. Despite this ultimate uncertainty, circumstantial evidence suggests that with normal cooperation motivation is not a problem in studies of children or adults. Two factors contribute to this acceptability: The muscle forces are relatively low at optimal velocity ($\sim$50% maximum isometric force), and the sensation of effort does not become apparent for about the first 15 s of an all-out maximal power output test.

In some forms of tests it is possible to apply an internal criterion, such as the linearity of the braking force/pedal rate relationship in a cycling exercise. Originally observed in adults (Sargeant et al., 1981; Vandewalle et al., 1985),

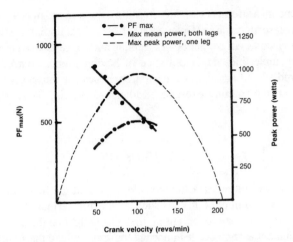

Figure 2.7 Maximal peak force (PFmax), maximal *mean* power (complete revolution of both legs), and maximal peak power (instantaneous power of one leg), in relation to pedaling rate from a series of isokinetic cycling tests performed by a 13-year-old boy. Maximal peak power is calculated from the inverse linear relationship of PFmax/velocity. The thick dashed line indicates the experimental range: the thin dashed line, the theoretical extrapolation. In the cycling exercise within the normal range the relationship of force to pedaling rate is linear (cf. Figure 2.2). (For a discussion of this see Sargeant et al., 1981.) *Note.* Data from Sargeant, Dolan, and Thorne, 1984.

this linearity has been subsequently confirmed in children (Figure 2.7). This observation allows the identification of low values compared within a series from the same individual, but it does not say anything about the status of the series as a whole.

Perhaps it is also comforting that changes in power output seen in children during training have been closely associated with increases in the active muscle mass (Sargeant et al., 1985). When increases in muscle size were taken into account, the reproducibility of tests over several months, during which motivational variation might be expected, was high (coefficient of variation = ±6%). This level of reproducibility is similar to that found in more detailed studies of adults (Coggan & Costill, 1984).

The extent to which power output is influenced by learning depends on the type of test chosen and the definition of *learning*. Most tests involve very common activities such as cycling, running, and jumping. Thus it might be assumed that relatively little margin exists for further learning of these skills that would improve performance. In repeated tests on adults on an isokinetic cycle ergometer, spaced out to avoid any direct muscle training effect, there was no systematic change in peak power output, and the coefficient of variation of the measurements was less than 6% (Sargeant et al., 1981). However, in a more unusual activity, maximal (10-s) sprints on a Monark cycle ergometer using *one* leg, the mean power output increased by 60% to 160% over 6 weeks. This massive increase occurred without any comparable changes in independent measurements of leg strength and power, muscle volume, or muscle cross-sectional area (Dolan et al., 1984). This finding is similar to that seen in many studies of weight/power training and suggests an element of neural learning. It underlines the importance of having proper control groups for training studies and additional criterion exercises for muscle power that are distinct from the training exercise (Rutherford, Greig, Sargeant, & Jones, 1986).

CONCLUSION

Short-term power output is a fundamental aspect of the functional capability of an individual (adult or child). As such, it is worth serious attention not only for its scientific interest, but because it may throw light on the nature of growth and development as they occur in normal muscle, with all the significance that this has for the study of disease. Furthermore, by focusing attention on short-term muscle function, researchers can redress the balance of interest, which for some years has been heavily focused on aerobic function.

CHALLENGES FOR FUTURE RESEARCH

A great deal of work still needs to be done in the area of human short-term power output, and this is especially true in studies of growth and development in children. The following are some major issues to consider:

- Few normative data exist for short-term power output in children, and existing data are sparse and cross-sectional. As yet no systematic long-term longitudinal data have been collected.

- Where data have been collected it is often difficult to make comparisons because of differences in technique and a failure to report important dimensional characteristics of the children studied (e.g., active muscle size).

- The phenomenon of the increase in short-term power output (standardized for body or muscle size) with age is not fully explained.

- There is a need to refine existing techniques and develop new ones to make meaningful estimates of changes in muscle dimensions and architecture associated with changes in power output.

- Some of the preceding points may derive useful data from carefully designed training studies. Until now, few studies have been conducted of the effect of training on short-term power in children.

- At present, very few published data exist on short-term power output from arm muscles in children.

REFERENCES

Asmussen, E., & Bøje, O. (1945). Body temperature and capacity for work. *Acta Physiologica Scandinavica, 107*, 33-37.

Asmussen, E., & Bonde-Petersen, F. (1974). Storage of elastic energy in skeletal muscle in man. *Acta Physiologica Scandinavica, 91*, 385-392.

Åstrand, P.O. (1952). *Experimental studies of physical working capacity in relation to sex and age.* Copenhagen: Munksgaard.

Ayalon, A., Inbar, O., & Bar-Or, O. (1974). Relationships among measurements of explosive strength and anaerobic power. In R.C. Nelson & C.A. Morehouse (Eds.), *International series on sport sciences: Vol. 1. Biomechanics IV* (pp. 572-577). Baltimore: University Park Press.

Bar-Or, O. (1987). The Wingate anaerobic test. An update on methodology, reliability and validity. *Sports Medicine* (New Zealand), *4*, 381-394.

Bassey, E.J., Dudley, B.R., & Pearson, M.B. (1985). The problem of resonance in isokinetic dynamometers. *Journal of Physiology, 361*, 7P.

Benedict, F.G., & Cathcart, E.P. (1913). *Muscular work: A metabolic study with special reference to the efficiency of the human body as a machine* (Report No. 187). Washington, DC: Carnegie Institute of Washington.

Bergh, U., & Ekblom, B. (1979). Influence of muscle temperature on maximal muscle strength and power output in human skeletal muscles. *Acta Physiologica Scandinavica, 107*, 33-37.

Blimkie, C.J.R., Roache, P., Hay, J.T., & Bar-Or, O. (1988). Anaerobic power of arms in teenage boys and girls: Relationship to lean tissue. *European Journal of Applied Physiology, 57*, 677-683..

Blix, M. (1906). *To the question of human working power.* Lund, Sweden: University Programme.

Bobbert, M.F., Hoek, E., van Ingen Schenau, G.J., Sargeant, A.J., & Schreurs, A.W. (1987). A model to demonstrate the power transporting role of bi-articular muscles. *Journal of Physiology, 387*, 24P.

Bouisset, S., Cnockaert, J.C., & Pertuzon, E. (1966). Sur la vitesse maximale de raccoucissement du muscle au court d'un mouvement monoarticulaire simple [Maximum speed of contraction of muscle in monoarticular movements]. *Journal of Physiology* (Paris), *58*, 474.

Caiozzo, V.J., & Kyle, C.R. (1980). The effect of external loading upon power output in stair climbing. *European Journal of Applied Physiology, 44*, 217-222.

Coggan, A.R., & Costill, D.L. (1984). Biological and technological variability of three anaerobic ergometer tests. *International Journal of Sports Medicine, 5*, 142-145.

Crielaard, J.M., & Pirnay, F. (1981). Anaerobic and aerobic power of top athletes. *European Journal of Applied Physiology, 47*, 295-300.

Cumming, G.R. (1973). Correlation of athletic performance and aerobic power in 12-17 year-old children with bone age, calf muscle, total body potassium, heart volume and two indices of anaerobic power. In O. Bar-Or (Ed.), *Pediatric work physiology* (pp. 109-134). Natanya: Wingate Institute.

Cumming, G.R., Hastman, J., McCort, J., & McCullough, S. (1980). High serum lactates do occur in young children after maximal work. *International Journal of Sports Medicine, 1*, 66-69.

Davies, C.T.M. (1971). Human power output in exercise of short duration in relation to body size and composition. *Ergonomics, 14*, 245-256.

Davies, C.T.M. (1985). Strength and mechanical properties of muscle in children and young adults. *Scandinavian Journal of Sports Science, 7*, 11-15.

Davies, C.T.M., Barnes, C., & Godfrey, S. (1972). Body composition and maximal exercise performance in children. *Human Biology, 44*, 195-214.

Davies, C.T.M., & Rennie, R. (1968). Human power output. *Nature, 217*, 770.

Davies, C.T.M., & Sargeant, A.J. (1974). Physiological responses to standardised arm work. *Ergonomics, 17*, 41-49.

Davies, C.T.M., & Sargeant, A.J. (1975). Effects of training on the physiological responses to one- and two-leg work. *Journal of Applied Physiology, 38*, 377-381.

Davies, C.T.M., Wemyss-Holden, J., & Young, K. (1984). Measurement of short term power output: Comparison between cycling and jumping. *Ergonomics, 27*, 285-296.

Davies, C.T.M., White, M.J., & Young, K. (1983). Muscle function in children. *European Journal of Applied Physiology, 52*, 111-114.

Davies, C.T.M., & Young, K. (1983). Effect of temperature on the contractile properties and muscle power of the triceps surae in humans. *Journal of Applied Physiology, 55*, 191-195.

Davies, C.T.M., & Young, K. (1984). Effects of external loading on short term power output in children and young male adults. European *Journal of Applied Physiology, 52*, 351-354.

de Koning, F.L., Binkhorst, R.A., Vos, J.A., & Van't Hof, M.A. (1985). The force velocity relationship of arm flexion in untrained males and females and arm-trained athletes. *European Journal of Applied Physiology, 54*, 89-94.

Dern, R.J., Levene, J.M., & Blair, H.A. (1947). Forces exerted at different velocities in human arm movements. *American Journal of Physiology, 151*, 415-437.

di Prampero, P.E., & Cerretelli, P. (1969). Maximal muscular power (aerobic and anaerobic) in African natives. *Ergonomics, 1*, 51-59.

Dolan, P., Greig, C.A., Grindrod, S., Narici, M., Rutherford, O., & Sargeant, A.J. (1984). Effect of fast and slow resistance training on maximal leg force and muscle size in man. *Journal of Physiology*, **354**, 100P.

Dotan, R., & Bar-Or, O. (1980). Climatic heat stress and performance in the Wingate anaerobic test. *European Journal of Applied Physiology*, **44**, 237-243.

Dotan, R., & Bar-Or. O. (1983). Load optimisation for the Wingate anaerobic test. *European Journal of Applied Physiology*, **51**, 409-417.

Elftman, M. (1940). Work done by muscle in running. *American Journal of Physiology*, **129**, 679.

Ericksson, B.O. (1972). Physical training, oxygen supply, and muscle metabolism in 11-13-year old boys. *Acta Physiologica Scandinavica*, (Suppl. 384).

Fenn, W.O. (1930). Frictional and kinetic factors in the work of sprint running. *American Journal of Physiology*, **92**, 583.

Fenn, W.O., & Marsh, B.S. (1935). Muscular force at different speeds of shortening. *Journal of Physiology*, **85**, 277-297.

Ferretti, G., Gussoni, M., di Prampero, P.E., & Cerretelli, P. (1987). Effects of exercise on maximal instantaneous muscular power of humans. *Journal of Applied Physiology*, **62**, 2288-2294.

Friden, J. (1983). Exercise-induced muscle soreness. *Umea University Medical Dissertations*. (New Series No. 105.)

Hill, A.V. (1922). The maximum work and mechanical efficiency of human muscles, and their most economical speed. *Journal of Physiology*, **56**, 19-41.

Hill, A.V. (1938). The heat of shortening and the dynamic constant of muscle. *Proceedings of the Royal Society of London*, **126**, 136-195.

Hill, A.V. (1970). *First and last experiments in muscle mechanics*. Cambridge, England: Cambridge University Press.

Inbar, O., & Bar-Or, O. (1975). The effects of intermittent warm-up on 7-9-year-old boys. *European Journal of Applied Physiology*, **34**, 81-89.

Inbar, O., & Bar-Or, O. (1986). Anaerobic characteristics of male children and adolescents. *Medicine and Science in Sports and Exercise*, **18**, 264-269.

Inbar, O., Dotan, R., Trousil, T., & Dvir, Z. (1983). The effect of bicycle crank length variation upon power performance. *Ergonomics*, **26**, 1139-1146.

Jones, D.A., Newham, D.J., Round, J.M., & Tolfree, S.E.J. (1986). Experimental muscle damage: Morphological changes in relation to other indices of damage. *Journal of Physiology*, **375**, 435-448.

Jones, P.R.M. (1970). *An application of physiological anthropometry*. Unpublished doctoral dissertation, University of Technology, Loughborough, England.

Jones, P.R.M., & Pearson, J. (1969). Anthropometric determination of leg fat and muscle plus bone volumes in young male and female adults. *Journal of Physiology*, **204**, 63-66P.

Katch, V.L, Weltman, A., Martin, R., & Gray, L. (1977). Optimal test characteristics for maximal anaerobic work on the bicycle ergometer. *Research Quarterly*, **48**, 319-327.

Kitagawa, L., Suzuki, M., & Miyashita, M. (1980). Anaerobic power output of young obese men: Comparison with non-obese men and the role of excess fat. *European Journal of Applied Physiology*, **43**, 229-234.

Lakomy, H.K.A. (1986). Measurement of work and power output using friction-loaded cycle ergometers. *Ergonomics*, **29**, 509-517.

Marechal, R., Pirnay, F., Crielaard, J.M., & Petit, J.M. (1979). *Influence de l'age sur la puissance anaerobic* [Effect of age on anaerobic power]. Paris: Economica. Paper presented at the Primier Colloque Medical International de Gymnastique, Strasbourg (1978, October).

Margaria, R., Aghemo, P., & Rovelli, E. (1966). Measurement of muscular power (anaerobic) in man. *Journal of Applied Physiology*, **21**, 1662-1664.

Margaria, R., di Prampero, P.E., Aghemo, P., Derevenco, P., & Mariani, M. (1971). Effect of steady-state exercise on maximal anaerobic power in man. *Journal of Applied Physiology*, **30**, 885-889.

McCarteney, N., Heigenhauser, G.J.F., Sargeant, A.J., & Jones, N.L. (1983). A constant velocity cycle ergometer for the study of dynamic muscle function. *Journal of Applied Physiology*, **55**, 212-217.

Narici, M.V., Roi, G.S., & Landoni, L. (1988). Force of knee extensor and flexor muscles and cross-sectional area determined by nuclear magnetic resonance imaging. *European Journal of Applied Physiology*, **57**, 39-44.

Newsholme, E.A., (1978). Substrate cycles: Their metabolic, energetic and thermic consequences in man. *Biochemical Society Symposia*, **43**, 183-205.

Nielsen, M., & Hansen, O. (1937). Maximal korperliche Arbeit bei Atmung O_2-reicher Luft. [Maximum physical work in O_2 enriched air]. *Skandinavisches Archiv für Physiologie*, **76**, 37-59.

Nonweiler, T.R.F. (1958). The work production of man: Studies on racing cyclists. *Journal of Physiology*, **141**, 8P.

Perrine, J.J., & Edgerton, V.R. (1978). Muscle force-velocity and power-velocity relationships under isokinetic loading. *Medicine and Science in Sports*, **10**, 159-166.

Pirnay, F., & Crielaard, J.M. (1979). Mesure de la puissance anaerobie alactique [Measurement of anaerobic alactic power]. *Medicine de Sport*, **53**, 13-16.

Ralston, H.J., Polissar, M.J., Inman, V.T., Close, J.A., & Feinstein, B. (1949). Dynamic features of human isolated voluntary muscle in isometric and free contractions. *Journal of Applied Physiology, 1*, 526-533.

Robinson, S. (1938). Experimental studies of physical fitness in relation to age. *Internationale Zeitschrift für Angewandte Physiologie, 10*, 251-323.

Rotstein, A., Dotan, R., Bar-Or, O., & Tenenbaum, G. (1986). Effect of training on anaerobic threshold, maximal aerobic power and anaerobic performance of preadolescent boys. *International Journal of Sports Medicine, 7*, 281-286.

Rutherford, O., Greig, C.A., Sargeant, A.J., & Jones, D.A. (1986). Strength training and power output—Transference effects in the human quadriceps muscle. *Journal of Sports Science, 4*, 101-107.

Sahlin, K. (1986). Metabolic changes limiting muscle performance. In B. Saltin (Ed.), *Biochemistry of exercise* (Vol. 6, pp. 323-344). Champaign, IL: Human Kinetics.

Sargeant, A.J. (1987). Effect of muscle temperature on leg extension force and short-term power output in humans. *European Journal of Applied Physiology, 56*, 693-698.

Sargeant, A.J., & Davies, C.T.M. (1977a). Limb volume, composition and maximum aerobic power output in relation to habitual preference in young male subjects. *Annals of Human Biology, 4*, 49-55.

Sargeant, A.J., & Davies, C.T.M. (1977b). The effects of disuse muscular atrophy on the forces generated in dynamic exercise. *Clinical Science and Molecular Medicine, 53*, 183-188.

Sargeant, A.J., Davies, C.T.M., Edwards, R.H.T., Maunder, C., & Young, A. (1977). Functional and structural changes following disuse of human muscle. *Clinical Science and Molecular Medicine, 52*, 337-342.

Sargeant, A.J., Dolan, P., & Young, A. (1984). Optimal velocity for maximal short-term power output in cycling. *International Journal of Sports Medicine, 5*, 124-125.

Sargeant, A.J., & Dolan, P. (1986). Optimal velocity of muscle contraction for short-term (anaerobic) power output in children and adults. In J. Rutenfranz, R. Mocellin, & F. Klimt (Eds.), *Children and Exercise* (Vol. 12, pp. 39-42). Champaign, IL: Human Kinetics.

Sargeant, A.J., & Dolan, P. (1987a). Effect of prior exercise on maximal short-term power output in man. *Journal of Applied Physiology: Respiratory, Environmental, and Exercise Physiology, 63*, 1475-1480.

Sargeant, A.J., & Dolan, P. (1987b). Human muscle function following prolonged eccentric exercise. *European Journal of Applied Physiology, 56*, 704-711.

Sargeant, A.J., Dolan, P., & Thorne, A. (1984). Isokinetic measurement of leg force and anaerobic power output in children. In J. Ilmarinen & I. Välimäki (Eds.), *Children and sport* (pp. 93-98). Berlin: Springer-Verlag.

Sargeant, A.J., Dolan, P., & Thorne, A. (1985). Effects of supplemental physical activity on body composition, aerobic and anaerobic power in 13-year-old boys. In R.A. Binkhorst, H.C.G. Kemper, & W.H.M. Saris (Eds.), *Children and exercise* (Vol. 11, pp. 135-139). Champaign, IL: Human Kinetics.

Sargeant, A.J., Hoinville, E., & Young, A. (1981). Maximum leg force and power output during short-term dynamic exercise. *Journal of Applied Physiology: Respiratory, Environmental, and Exercise Physiology, 51*(5), 1175-1182.

Sargent, D.A. (1921). The physical test of a man. *American Physical Education Review, 26*, 188-194.

Sargent, L.W. (1924). Some observations on the Sargent test of neuromuscular efficiency. *American Physical Education Review, 29*, 47-56.

Steplock, D.A., Veicsteinas, A., & Mariani, M. (1971). Maximal aerobic and anaerobic power and stroke volume of the heart in a subalpine population. *Internationale Zeitschrift für Angewandte Physiologie, 29*, 203-214.

Thomas, D.O., White, M.J., Sagar, G., & Davies, C.T.M. (1987). Electrically evoked plantar flexor torque in males. *Journal of Applied Physiology, 63*, 1499-1503.

Thorstensonn, A., Grimby, G., & Karlsson, J. (1976). Force-velocity relationships and fiber composition in human knee extensor muscle. *Journal of Applied Physiology, 40*, 12-16.

Tuttle, W.W. (1949). Effect of physical training on capacity to do work as measured by the bicycle ergometer. *Journal of Applied Physiology, 2*, 393-398.

Unna, P.J.H. (1946). Limits of effective human power. *Nature, 158*, 560-561.

Vandewalle, H., Peres, G., Heller, J., & Monod, H. (1985). All out anaerobic capacity test on cycle ergometers. *European Journal of Applied Physiology, 54*, 222-229.

Vandewalle, H., Peres, G., Heller, J., Panel, J., & Monod, H. (1987). Force-velocity relationship and maximal power on a cycle ergometer. Correlation with the height of a vertical jump. *European Journal of Applied Physiology, 56*, 650-656.

Vandewalle, H., Peres, G., & Monod, H. (1984). Puissance maximale et capacité de travail pour des exercices de brève durée [Maximum power and capacity for short duration exercise]. *Journal of Physiology (Paris), 79*, 36A-37A.

Vandewalle, H., Peres, G., & Monod, H. (1987). Standard anaerobic exercise tests. *Sports Medicine* (New Zealand), **4**, 268-289.

Wickiewicz, T.L., Roy, R.R., Powell, P.L., Perrine, J.J., & Edgerton, V.R. (1984). Muscle architecture and force velocity relations in humans. *Journal of Applied Physiology,* **57**, 435-443.

Wilkie, D.R. (1950). The relation between force and velocity in human muscle. *Journal of Physiology,* **110**, 249-280.

Wilkie, D.R. (1960). Man as a source of mechanical power. *Ergonomics,* **3**, 1-8.

Winter, D.A., Wells, R.P., & Orr, G.W. (1981). Errors in the use of isokinetic dynamometers. *European Journal of Applied Physiology,* **46**, 397-408.

3

Development of the Oxygen Transport System in Normal Children

Dan M. Cooper
Harbor-UCLA Medical Center

As children grow and develop, the gas exchange system (i.e., heart, lung, blood, and vessels) must change in such a way that increasingly large metabolic demands, particularly those imposed by physical exercise, can be appropriately matched to oxygen delivery. Growth is a homeostatic process—one in which certain functions and components of the organism undergo significant change while others remain largely unchanged. For example, whereas the maximal oxygen consumption of 18-year-old teenagers is, on average, about three times as large as values obtained in 6-year-old boys, the mechanical work efficiency remains 28% in both groups (Cooper, Weiler-Ravell, Whipp, & Wasserman, 1984a). Thus certain aspects of the gas exchange system are *regulated* as normal growth proceeds. Determining how the growth of the oxygen transport is controlled during childhood requires a knowledge of the regulated variables. This chapter reviews the theoretical and experimental approaches that have been used to identify these regulated variables.

The development of models useful for understanding cardiorespiratory growth in children is becoming increasingly important for several practical reasons. In considering children with chronic disease or disability, researchers must develop reasonable physical activity programs that take into account not only the immediate limitations of the child, but also the long-term effects of inactivity on the growth process itself. For healthy children, the popular concern for physical fitness (Toufexis, 1987) has focused attention on the degree to which children ought to participate in physical fitness programs or competitive athletes. Thus our challenge is clear—to develop rational guidelines that define too much as well as too little physical activity for both normal and disabled children. Finally, although the utility of exercise testing in adult medicine for the assessment of heart and lung disease is well established (Wasserman, Hansen, Sue, & Whipp, 1987), such testing in pediatric settings is infrequently used on a clinical basis. By understanding more fully how exercise responses are related to the growth process itself, we can determine appropriate uses of exercise testing in children.

THEORETICAL CONSIDERATIONS

Allometric Equations and the Dimensionless Mass Exponent

A major component of growth in children is the obvious increase in body size, and the relationship between body size and metabolic function has been a central area of investigation for comparative physiologists. At the core of this research is the idea that constraints on metabolic function (e.g., thermoregulation, exercise responses) are imposed by physical properties related to body size and structure. Attempts have been made to develop unifying theories and models that would predict how a particular metabolic function changes with body size (Schmidt-Nielsen, 1972). Central to these efforts is the concept of *biological similarity* (Gunther, 1975; Rosen, 1983), which holds that because all living things (unicellular and multicellular) are subjected to similar physical and chemical influences from the environment, the structure and function of animals, irrespective of size, can be studied from first principles (e.g., laws of mechanics, diffusion). For example, despite the fact that an elephant is roughly a million times the size of a mouse, the diffusion of oxygen across tissue membranes in both animals is ultimately governed by the same set of physical principles, and the functional capabilities of the cardiorespiratory systems of both animals are constrained by these laws. *Allometric equations* are used to relate physiologic function to body size (Gould, 1966). These equations commonly appear in the following form:

$$q \propto a \cdot M^b \qquad (1)$$

where q indicates a metabolic function (e.g., maximal O_2 uptake), M is a dimension-related parameter (usually body mass), a is the mass coefficient, and b is the dimensionless mass exponent or the scaling factor.

Theoretical Predictions of the Dimensionless Mass Exponent

One of the first theories used to derive the dimensionless mass exponent was the *surface area law* (Gray, 1981). This principle held that metabolic rate in mammals is determined by the need to maintain temperature homeostasis. Heat production must equal heat loss, the latter being proportional to the surface area-to-body-mass ratio of the animal. Because this ratio is proportional to body mass to the power of 2/3, it was reasoned that basal oxygen uptake ($\dot{V}O_2$), heat production, and other metabolic rates (including those during exercise) must also scale to body mass to the 2/3 power. It is interesting that the notion that metabolic function in children scales to body surface area is still quite prevalent. Drug dosages, cancer chemotherapy protocols, and fluid replacement regimens are often based on surface area despite the fact that no direct measurement of surface area is available in living children.

An alternative construct was presented by Hill (1950), a pioneering comparative physiologist of this century, who expanded the concept of *geometric similarity* to predict the scaling factor relating $\dot{V}O_2$ to body weight. Hill argued that in animals of different body mass, the proportion of the body's components (i.e., limbs, trunk) remained the same despite differences in size. Thus, for example, if limb *length* in one animal was twice that of another, the *diameter* of the larger animal's limb would also be twice as large. He further assumed that muscle force per muscle cross-sectional area (i.e., stress) was independent of the overall body size. Finally, he proposed that the maximal oxygen uptake ($\dot{V}O_2$max) would depend on the product of cross-sectional area of the limb and the peak stress. From these assumptions about muscle strength and body geometry in animals of different sizes, Hill predicted that the maximal oxygen uptake should scale to the 2/3 power of body mass for the following reasons:

$$\text{Peak muscle force} \propto \text{cross-sectional area} \qquad (2)$$

$$\text{Cross-sectional area} \propto \ell^2 \qquad (3)$$
$$\text{where } \ell \text{ is a linear body dimension}$$

$$\text{Body weight (W)} \propto \ell^3 \qquad (4)$$
$$\text{by geometric similarity}$$

$$\text{Peak muscle force} \propto W^{2/3} \qquad (5)$$

$$\dot{V}O_2\text{max} \propto \text{peak muscle force } W^{2/3} \qquad (6)$$

Recently, McMahon (1973, 1984) proposed the concept of *elastic similarity* to account for the observed relationship between body mass and maximal oxygen consumption in mature animals of widely different sizes. This theory holds that the similarity of many mammals lies not in their geometric characteristics, but rather in their need to maintain structural integrity in response to forces produced around joints and limbs resulting from terrestrial locomotion. By McMahon's reasoning, the elastic properties of the animal, those involved in the physics of bending and buckling as the animal moves, are central. Despite changes in body size, the elastic properties of the animal must be maintained so that joints do not buckle during terrestrial locomotion. The predictions of this theory are different from those of geometric similarity or the surface area law. In animals of different size, the length of a limb will not scale in direct proportion to its diameter (i.e., to the power of 1), but rather to the power of 2/3. As a result, the cross-sectional area is proportional to the 3/4 power of body mass, and $\dot{V}O_2$max scales to the 3/4 power of weight as well.

Relationship Between Theory and Observation

What, in fact, do the data show? One of the well-known collections of such data is the "mouse-to-elephant" curve shown in Figure 3.1 (Kleiber, 1947,

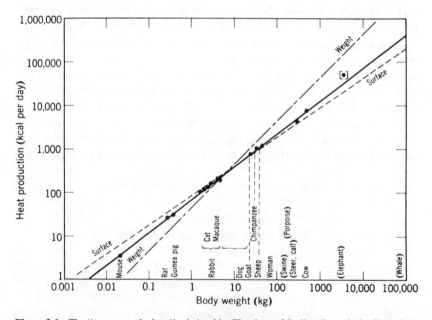

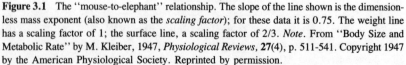

Figure 3.1 The "mouse-to-elephant" relationship. The slope of the line shown is the dimensionless mass exponent (also known as the *scaling factor*); for these data it is 0.75. The weight line has a scaling factor of 1; the surface line, a scaling factor of 2/3. *Note.* From "Body Size and Metabolic Rate" by M. Kleiber, 1947, *Physiological Reviews, 27*(4), p. 511-541. Copyright 1947 by the American Physiological Society. Reprinted by permission.

1975). This represents the basal metabolic rates of a variety of animals plotted against body weight. The mass exponent of this relationship is 3/4, and not the 2/3 power predicted by the surface area law or Hill's geometric similarity. Criticism of the mouse-to-elephant curve has arisen because the data presented in it were obtained from many different sources using a wide variety of techniques. More recent work by Taylor, Weibel, and co-workers concentrated on maximal oxygen uptakes of a range of mature animals of different sizes in Africa (Taylor, Maloiy, et al., 1981; Taylor & Weibel, 1981; Weibel et al., 1981). The results of their studies are shown in Table 3.1. Note that the dimensionless mass exponent was not 2/3, nor was it in all cases 3/4 (that predicted by McMahon for pure elastic similarity).

Table 3.1   Scaling Factors Relating Metabolic Function and Body Mass During Exercise in Animals and Human Subjects ($q = a \cdot M^b$).

	Scaling factor (b)	95% confidence interval
Wild animals	0.793	0.754-0.833
Domestic animals	0.764	0.603-0.845
Wild and domestic animals	0.769	0.736-0.801
Boys and girls ($\dot{V}O_2$max)	1.01	0.90-1.11
Boys and girls (anaerobic threshold)	0.92	0.80-1.02

Note. Animal data from Taylor et al., 1981; human subject data from Cooper, Mellins, and Mansell, 1981.

Much debate has recently been generated concerning the physiological significance of the dimensionless mass exponent. Heusner (1982a, 1982b, 1983) has argued that the scaling factor, 3/4, used in considering interspecies relationships between size and function may actually be artifactual. A number of studies, in fact, demonstrate that within some species (e.g., guinea pigs), the scaling factor is 2/3 (Wilkie, 1977). Feldman and McMahon (1983) countered Heusner's argument with a statistical analysis of simple and parallel regression that outlines the different mathematical approach needed to compare intra- with interspecies data. These authors assert that

> both mass exponents, 2/3 (intra-species) and 3/4 (inter-species), may have biological meaning. Perhaps genetic instructions require that the shapes of animals be maintained constant within species, but the shapes of related animals of grossly different size (the dik-dik and the eland, for example) have been allowed by evolution to diverge in ways dictated by the influence of gravity and inertia. There is no reason

based on thermodynamics or any other science why the mass exponent 3/4 should not describe the inter-species rising metabolic rate of mammals. The statistics say the relation is there, and we are challenged to understand it. (p. 159)

Various investigators have attempted to use allometric analyses in studying growth of the oxygen transport system in children (Asmussen & Heeboll-Nielsen, 1955; Von Dobeln, Åstrand, & Bergstrom, 1967). In our own laboratory, 109 normal subjects ranging in age from 6 to 18 performed progressive exercise using a ramp-type input and breath-to-breath measurement of gas exchange (Cooper et al., 1984a). The measured dimensionless mass exponent relating $\dot{V}O_2$max and body weight in our sample population is shown in Table 3.1. Note that the scaling factors for both $\dot{V}O_2$max and the anaerobic threshold were not statistically different from 1.0. The implication of these findings is that $\dot{V}O_2$max normalized to body weight (i.e., $\dot{V}O_2$max • kg^{-1}) would not change with increasing body size in children (Figure 3.2). Interestingly, the same scaling factor was found in a reanalysis of the data collected by Åstrand (1952) also shown in Table 3.1.

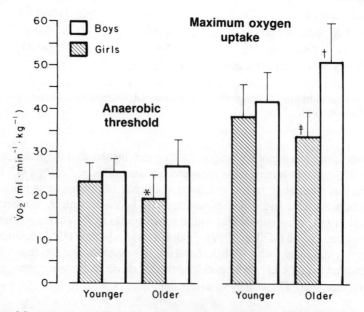

Figure 3.2 Anaerobic threshold (AT) and the maximal oxygen uptake, normalized to body weight, in 109 normal children. Although there were no significant differences between the younger and older children for the normalized AT or $\dot{V}O_2$max, there were gender-related differences: Older girls had significantly lower ATs than the other groups ($p < .05$ by ANOVA and modified t test); older boys had the highest normalized $\dot{V}O_2$max ($p < .05$ by ANOVA and modified t test) than did the other groups; and older girls had significantly lower normalized $\dot{V}O_2$max (p × .05 ANOVA and modified t test).

How can the discrepancy between the observed dimensionless mass exponents and theoretical predictions be reconciled? The data demonstrate that neither the surface area law nor geometric similarity adequately describes structure-function relationships in terrestrial mammals. McMahon's principle of elastic similarity yields the most accurate prediction. It is tempting to infer, then, from these data, that the process of locomotion per se will influence the growth of gas transport systems during growth in children. One might expect the relationship between metabolic function and structure to differ greatly when comparing infants in the first years of life to older children in whom physical activity is a routine part of daily living. In fact, recent work by Zeltner and co-workers (Zeltner & Burri, 1987; Zeltner, Caduff, Gehr, Pfenninger, & Burri, 1987) on lung growth supports this hypothesis (see next section).

Despite the accuracy of elastic similarity in predicting the scaling factor of mature mammals, the data show that the relationship between metabolic function and body mass during growth in children is governed by a different set of principles from that which determines structure-function relationships in mature animals of different sizes. $\dot{V}O_2$max (and the anaerobic threshold) scale to body mass to the power of 1, in contrast to the results obtained in mature mammals. Additional analyses of the data in children allow some interesting insights into the growth process itself.

By the principle of geometric similarity, body height should scale to body mass to the 1/3 power, and, in fact, this is precisely what we found in our sample of 109 children. But despite this agreement between the theory and observation in children, the $\dot{V}O_2$max in children scaled to the power of 1 and not the 2/3 predicted by geometric similarity. A solution to this discrepancy can be found by challenging an assumption of Hill's model and of elastic similarity, namely, that muscle stress is independent of body size. If there existed a maturational process within the muscles themselves such that they can generate greater force for their cross-sectional area as children grow, then the discrepancy between theory and observation would be eliminated. Interestingly, observations made by Asmussen and Heeboll-Nielsen (1955) support the concept that muscles change not only in size during the growth process, but in their intrinsic strength as well. Further work needs to be done to determine precisely how dimensional analysis can be used to characterize cardiorespiratory responses to exercise in children.

The data show that the growth process represents a unique relationship between structure and function in biology. Applying the type of analysis previously outlined may allow us to gain nonintuitive information about how oxygen transport is linked to size during growth.

Allometry, Morphometry, and Human Lung Growth

A fascinating example of how such analysis can be used to understand the growth of the O_2 transport system was presented recently by Zeltner and co-workers (Zeltner & Burri, 1987; Zeltner et al., 1987). Using autopsy specimens from children aged 26 days to 5 years and from adults who had died of nonpulmonary causes, the authors attempted to relate diffusing capacity for O_2 to the growth in alveolar volume. Morphometric techniques were used to estimate the diffusing capacity for O_2. Two separate phases of lung growth were identified. In the first phase, lasting from birth to approximately 18 months, the capillary volume increased with body mass to the power of 2.114, whereas the parenchymal airspace volume increased with a scaling factor of 1.155. In Phase 2, both of these rates of increase slowed considerably (scaling factors of 0.997 for capillary volume and 1.059 for parenchymal airspace volume). It is noteworthy that this change in growth of a critical aspect of the O_2 transport system occurred in the same period when infants are usually becoming fully bipedal and independent in locomotion. Additional investigations are clearly necessary to assess the changes in the gas exchange system that occur with the onset of walking in children.

Zeltner and co-workers also found that the diffusing capacity for O_2 increased with body mass to the 1.15 power (the latter being significantly different from 1.0; see Figure 3.3) and noted that the diffusing capacity increased more rapidly

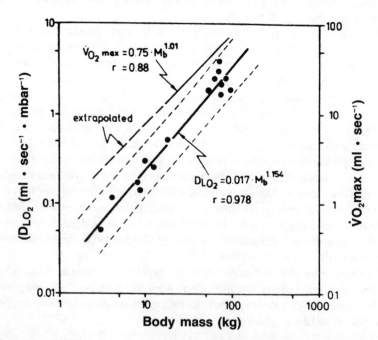

Figure 3.3 Allometric plot of the morphometric pulmonary O_2 diffusing capacity (DL_{O_2}) of seven children and eight adults in comparison with maximal O_2 uptake ($\dot{V}O_2$max) and the 95% confidence band for DL_{O_2} (dashed lines). (The allometric relationship of $\dot{V}O_2$max was calculated from the data presented by Cooper et al., 1984.) *Note*. From "The Postnatal Development and Growth of the Human Lung: 1. Morphometry" by T.B. Zeltner and P.H. Burri, 1987, *Respiration Physiology*, **67**, pp. 247-267. Copyright 1987 by Elsevier. Reprinted by permission.

in children than did the $\dot{V}O_2$max. A similar observation was made in inter-species comparisons of mammals (Weibel, 1984). Weibel et al. (1981) suggested that the relatively greater diffusing capacities were necessary to compensate for larger acinar pathway lengths in the bigger animals. However, as Zeltner points out in his work, little attention has yet been paid to the discordant scaling in human beings.

INTENSIVE AND EXTENSIVE PROPERTIES OF CARDIORESPIRATORY GROWTH

Concepts

In a recent analysis of the physiological significance of allometric relationships, Heusner (1983) suggested that properties of animals can be divided into two groups: *extensive properties*—those that are dependent on body mass, such as length, surface area, or energy metabolism; and *intensive properties*—those that are largely independent of body mass, such as density, temperature, or pressure. Although extensive properties describe the *quantitative* aspects of the animal, intensive properties are essentially *qualitative* in nature, often being ratios of extensive properties. Heusner suggested that the mass coefficient of allometric equations (*a* in Equation 1) is possibly a species-specific intensive property because it is defined as

$$a = q/M^b \qquad (7)$$

representing the quotient of two extensive properties.

Heusner presented an interesting analogy to illustrate the meaning of qualitative versus quantitative properties. Consider, for example, the relationship between the surface area (SA) and volume (V) of a sphere and a cube. For the cube, $SA = 6 \cdot V^{2/3}$, whereas for the sphere, $SA = 4.84 \cdot V^{2/3}$. Thus it appears that even though both the sphere and the cube have the identical dimensionless mass exponent of 2/3, the qualitative difference between the sphere and the cube is confirmed by the different values of *a*. Heusner went on to consider the danger inherent in comparing animals of different intensive characteristics, where one could reach the conclusion that some animals have values for *a* that are *less than* 4.84, this being geometrically impossible (Figure 3.4). In looking at Figure 3.4, one sees that a line can be drawn from points on one line (O) to the other (□) and this line(dashed) will have a slope other than 2/3. The intercept of this line is less than point A, but there is no form that can have a smaller surface area to volume ratio than does a sphere. Heusner has nicely demonstrated how differences in qualitative properties (in this case, the geometrical form) can profoundly affect the interpretation of quantitative properties.

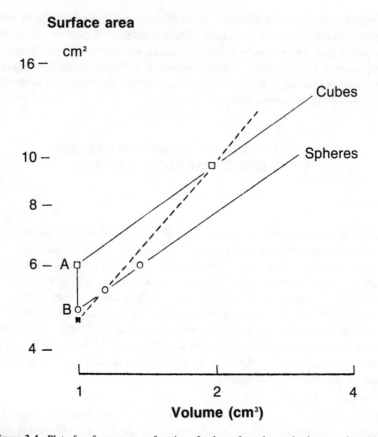

Figure 3.4 Plot of surface area as a function of volume for cubes and spheres on logarithmic scales, showing the scaling factor (in this case, the slope of each line) to be 2/3. Points A and B represent the y-intercepts: the surface area of a cube and sphere of unit mass, respectively. *Note*. From "Body Size, Energy Metabolism, and the Lungs" by A.A. Heusner, 1983, *Journal of Applied Physiology*, **54**, p. 868. Copyright 1983 by the American Physiological Society. Adapted by permission.

Extensive Properties of Cardiorespiratory Growth

Much has been written about the extensive properties related to exercise in children and how these properties change with growth (Table 3.2). In particular, Godfrey (1974), Bar-Or (1983), and Cunningham, Paterson, and Blimkie (1984) have written excellent reviews. An interesting extensive property of cardiorespiratory growth, and one that may have particular clinical relevance, is the relationship between $\dot{V}O_2$ and heart rate during exercise (Cooper, Weiler-Ravell, Whipp, & Wasserman, 1984b). These two factors are related by the Fick equation:

$$\dot{V}O_2 = SV \cdot HR \cdot (a\text{-}\bar{v})O_2 \text{ difference} \qquad (8)$$

where SV is stroke volume and $(a-\bar{v})O_2$ difference is the arteriovenous oxygen content difference. Because stroke volume is clearly an extensive property (i.e., it is directly related to the size of the heart) and the arteriovenous O_2 difference is intensive (i.e., it is related to the ratio of cellular O_2 consumption and blood flow), one would expect the relationship between $\dot{V}O_2$ and heart rate to be highly size dependent and to reflect the ability of the organism to extract oxygen per heart beat.

Table 3.2   Examples of Extensive and Intensive Properties of the Gas Exchange Response to Exercise in Children

Extensive properties	Intensive properties
$\dot{V}O_2$max	$\Delta\dot{V}O_2/\Delta WR$
$\dot{V}_E$max	$\Delta\dot{V}_E/\Delta VCO_2$
Anaerobic threshold	$\tau\dot{V}O$, $\tau\dot{V}CO$, $\tau\dot{V}_E$
$\Delta\dot{V}O_2/\Delta HR$	Lung mixing efficiency

The relationship between $\dot{V}O_2$ and heart rate during progressive exercise is shown in Figure 3.5 for an 8-year-old boy and a 17-year-old male teenager. The slope (designated as "M" in the figure, given as $\Delta\dot{V}O_2/\Delta HR$) is related to, but not the same as, *the O_2-pulse*, the latter being the ratio of the absolute value of $\dot{V}O_2$ divided by heart rate at any point during exercise ($\dot{V}O_2/HR$). The slope (M) increases with body weight in both boys and girls, although more rapidly in boys (as shown in Figure 3.6), and the dimensionless mass exponent for this relationship was 1.07 (not significantly different from 1.0). The data imply that the ability of children to extract O_2 per heart beat during exercise increases in direct proportion to body weight. Cardiorespiratory and musculoskeletal systems are integrated so that oxygen flow during exercise is optimized to meet the energy requirements of the muscle cells despite the changes in body size. In adults, the relationship between $\dot{V}O_2$ and heart rate during exercise is markedly affected by cardiac disease and is a clinically useful tool for diagnostic purposes (Wasserman et al., 1987). Figure 3.7 shows the results of a progressive exercise test for a 43-year-old man suffering from mitral insufficiency. As cardiac function diminishes, the heart becomes functionally smaller and the relationship between $\dot{V}O_2$ and heart rate assumes the characteristics of younger children. Much work needs to be done in children on the $\dot{V}O_2$—heart rate relationship during disease as well as to establish the effect of physical training.

Finally, the data show (Figure 3.6) marked differences of the $\dot{V}O_2$—heart rate relationship (m) between boys and girls. The observation of significant

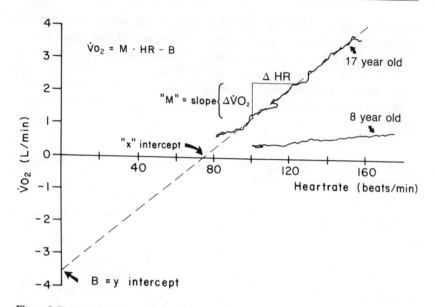

Figure 3.5 The relationship between $\dot{V}O_2$ and HR during progressive exercise in an 8- and a 17-year-old subject. *Note*. From "Oxygen Uptake and Heart Rate During Exercise as a Function of Growth in Children" by D.M. Cooper, D. Weiler-Ravell, B.J. Whipp, and K. Wasserman, 1984, *Pediatric Research*, **18**, p. 846. Copyright 1984 by Williams & Wilkins. Reprinted by permission.

gender-related differences in cardiorespiratory responses to exercise is well established for the $\dot{V}O_2$max and the anaerobic threshold (Figure 3.2; Åstrand, 1952; Bar-Or, 1983; Cooper et al., 1984a, 1984b; Godfrey, 1974). Whether these differences are related to iron deficiency anemia (more prevalent in teenage girls than boys), general levels of fitness, endocrinological factors, or intrinsic properties of muscle is not yet clear. Several lines of evidence suggest that the relationship between cardiorespiratory and musculoskeletal growth is the same in boys and girls and that differences between boys and girls are related to size alone or to differences in general fitness. Davies, Barnes, and Godfrey (1972) related $\dot{V}O_2$max to muscle calf volume rather than body weight and found that gender-related differences disappeared. We examined the relationship between the O_2 pulse (at 140 beats $\bullet$ min^{-1}) and body weight in boys and girls (Figure 3.8). As can be seen, distinct differences between boys and girls are present; however, when the O_2 pulse data were plotted as a function of the subjects' anaerobic threshold (AT) rather than body weight, the gender differences were eliminated. It appears that from a functional point of view, the integration of cardiorespiratory and musculoskeletal growth is the same in boys and girls.

In large part, the focus on extensive properties results from the relative ease of their measurement. However, there are also theoretical grounds for studying

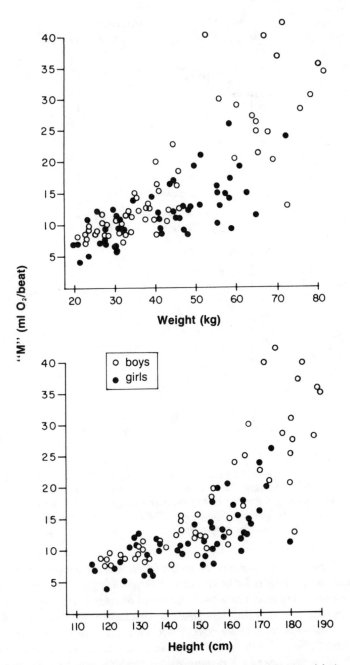

Figure 3.6 The slope (M) of the $\dot{V}O_2$—HR relationship as a function of body weight (top panel) and height (bottom panel) in the study population. *Note.* From ''Oxygen Uptake and Heart Rate During Exercise as a Function of Growth in Children'' by D.M. Cooper, D. Weiler-Ravell, B.J. Whipp, and K. Wasserman, 1984, *Pediatric Research,* **18,** p. 848. Copyright 1984 by Williams & Wilkins. Reprinted by permission.

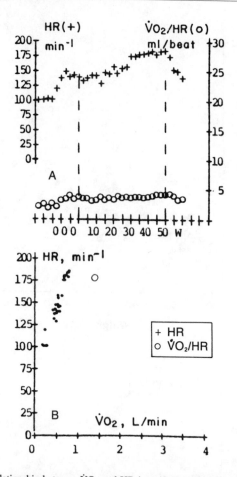

Figure 3.7 The relationship between $\dot{V}O_2$ and HR in a 43-year-old man suffering from mitral insufficiency: HR as a function of power in watts (W) (A) and HR as a function of $\dot{V}O_2$ (B). *Note*. From *Principles of Exercise Testing and Interpretation* (pp. 138-139) by K. Wasserman, J.E. Hansen, D.Y. Sue, and B.J. Whipp, 1987, Philadelphia: Lea & Febiger. Copyright 1987 by Lea & Febiger. Adapted by permission.

body-size-dependent parameters such as the maximal oxygen uptake. Most notable among these is the theory of *symmorphosis* (Taylor & Weibel, 1981), which attempts to model how the structure of oxygen delivery systems differs in mammals of widely different sizes. By this theory, the formation of structural elements is regulated to satisfy but not exceed the requirements of the functional system. Taylor and Weibel have taken these requirements to mean maximal capabilities of the system, such as the $\dot{V}O_2$max. The theory predicts that all elements of the O_2 transport system are designed to match this maximal demand; hence, one might predict the pattern of muscle capillarization, the cellular mitochondrial density, and the levels of oxidative enzymes.

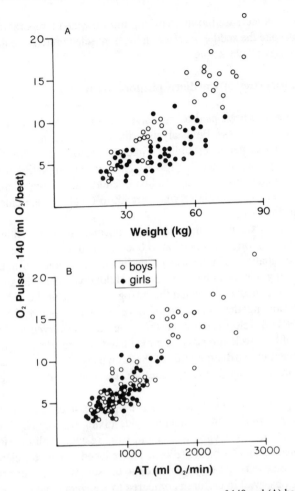

Figure 3.8 The relationship between O_2 pulse at a heart rate of 140 and (A) body weight, and (B) the anaerobic threshold (AT) in boys and girls. *Note.* From "Oxygen Uptake and Heart Rate During Exercise as a Function of Growth in Children" by D.M. Cooper, D. Weiler-Ravell, B.J. Whipp, and K Wasserman, 1984, *Pediatric Research,* **18,** p. 850. Copyright 1984 by Williams & Wilkins. Reprinted by permission.

Cooper et al. (1984b) proposed an alternative theoretical approach. Maximal efforts are rarely required in the daily lives of animals or children. Moreover, apparent redundancies in function occur in a number of physiological systems (e.g., liver). Far more important for the organism than maximal efforts is the ability to rapidly change from one level of energy expenditure to another. The transition from rest to exercise, or from one work rate to another, requires a highly integrated physiological response during which cellular homeostasis must be maintained despite large and rapid changes in cellular O_2 uptake and CO_2 production. Moreover, blood pressure must be maintained at the same time that flow is increased to the working muscles, and temperature must be controlled despite the sudden increase in local muscle temperature that accompanies increases in work rate.

Intensive Properties of Cardiorespiratory Growth

Little attention has been paid to intensive properties and how these change during the growth process. But analysis of these properties has already yielded new information as well as providing clinically acceptable methods of assessing exercise responses in children (Table 3.2). Intensive properties of the cardiorespiratory system can be readily studied in children. During exercise, these properties are easily identifiable when breath-to-breath measurements of gas exchange are available.

Consider, for example, lung growth in normal children. Although lung volume changes in direct proportion to body mass in children ranging in age from 6 to 18, analysis of intensive properties of lung function indicates that qualitative changes in the lungs occur during childhood. Using the single-breath oxygen test, a maneuver in which the nitrogen content of the exhaled gas is measured following the inhalation of pure oxygen, Cooper, Mellins, and Mansell (1981) developed the concept of the *mixing efficiency*. This serves as an index of how well atmospheric air is mixed with resident gas in the lung. It is determined by elastic qualities of the lung as well as by the relative size of airways and airspaces. It can, therefore, be seen as an intrinsic property of the lung.

The mixing efficiency was found to increase progressively with height (Figure 3.9) and age in normal children. Interestingly, mixing was actually less efficient when the inhalation of oxygen was begun from residual volume (RV) rather than functional residual capacity (FRC). The reduced mixing efficiency results in lower alveolar PO_2 and may be related to the somewhat lower arterial PO_2 values often observed in children compared to teenagers and adults (Cooper, Hyman, et al., 1985). During exercise, when respiratory frequency is markedly increased and tidal breaths begin at lung volumes below the subject's FRC, the reduced mixing efficiency of younger children may impair pulmonary gas exchange. Little is known at present about the efficiency of mixing inspired and resident gas during exercise in either healthy children or those with pulmonary disease.

The ratio of the increase in oxygen uptake to the increase in power output during a progressive exercise protocol is an example of an intensive property of cardiorespiratory growth during exercise. This measures how muscle metabolism is coupled with mechanical work (its inverse, with appropriate correction factors for metabolic fuel mix, is the work efficiency; Wasserman et al., 1987). If muscle cell energy metabolism were independent of the animal's size (a reasonable assumption), then body size per se would not affect this ratio. In fact, no such differences have been observed in children of different ages and sizes (Cooper et al., 1984a). In general, one can use observed differ-

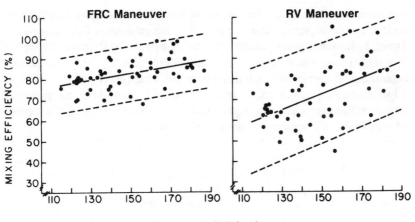

Figure 3.9 Mixing efficiency (means, solid lines; ± SD, dashed lines) as a function of height in 54 normal children for the FRC and RV maneuvers. *Note*. From "Changes in Distribution of Ventilation With Lung Growth" by D.M. Cooper, R.B. Mellins, and A.L. Mansell, 1981, *Journal of Applied Physiology*, **51**, p. 702. Copyright 1981 by The American Physiological Society. Reprinted by permission.

ences in intensive properties to test whether qualitative differences in function exist between adults and children, or among children of varying size and age. Other intensive properties during exercise, such as the ratio of ventilation and CO_2 production and the response characteristics of gas exchange at the onset of exercise, are discussed in the next section.

Heusner (1982a, 1982b) has argued that, by ignoring the differences between the intensive, qualitative properties that occur among animals of different species, researchers have reached false conclusions about the relationship between structure and function. His approach has particular relevance to studying metabolic function in children. The growth process is not uniform in either rate or development. Analysis of the intensive and extensive properties of growth during specific periods (e.g., the relationship between $\dot{V}O_2$max and body weight in the prepubertal and pubertal periods) may yield new insight into how the metabolic demand changes relative to body size and, ultimately, how the O_2 transport system must change to meet these demands. Heusner's analysis also highlights problems inherent to cross-sectional versus longitudinal study designs in populations of children.

DYNAMIC GAS EXCHANGE RESPONSES TO EXERCISE

Time Constant for $\dot{V}O_2$ at the Onset of Exercise

Techniques have been developed to analyze the *dynamic* responses of gas exchange to various inputs of metabolic demand, using breath-to-breath measurements (Beaver, Lamarra, & Wasserman, 1981; Lamarra, 1982). These techniques allow precise characterization of the responses. For example, in Figure 3.10, $\dot{V}O_2$ is plotted against time during a transition from rest to exercise in teenagers and children. It is important to note that the data represent the superimposed average of six transitions at the same power output in each of 10 subjects. Respiratory noise virtually precludes the accurate estimation of response characteristics from single transitions, and the averaging of a number of transitions is a standard technique for noise reduction.

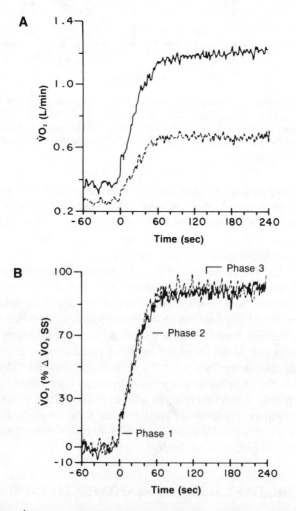

Figure 3.10 $\dot{V}O_2$ response kinetics at the onset (time D) of constant work rate exercise from 10 teenagers (solid lines) and from 10 7- to 10-year-old children (dashed lines). *Note*. From "Kinetics of Oxygen Uptake at the Onset of Exercise as a Function of Growth in Children" by D.M. Cooper, C. Berry, N. Lamarra, and K. Wasserman, 1985, *Journal of Applied Physiology, 59*, p.214. Copyright 1985 by The American Physiological Society. Reprinted by permission.

Three distinct phases have been identified in the $\dot{V}O_2$ response to exercise (Wasserman, Whipp, & Davis, 1981; Figure 3.10). Phase 1 is the *cardiodynamic* phase and represents the rapid increase in VO_2 commonly observed in the first 20 s of exercise. Current thinking holds that the Phase 1 response is tied to the sudden increase in cardiac output at the onset of exercise (Whipp & Ward, 1982). Moreover, it has been postulated that this increase is directly related to changes in the stroke volume. It is assumed that the blood returning to the heart in the first seconds of the transition (i.e., blood squeezed from the working muscles before additional O_2 has been extracted) has the same PO_2 as prior to the onset of exercise. By the Fick equation (Equation 8), if the $(a-\bar{v})O_2$ difference is constant, then changes in SV can be calculated from direct measurements of $\dot{V}O_2$ and HR.

Phase 2 of the response has been shown to be well described by an exponential equation of the following form:

$$\Delta\dot{V}O_2(t) = \Delta\dot{V}O_2(ss) \bullet (1 - e^{-t/\tau}) \qquad (9)$$

where $\Delta\dot{V}O_2(t)$ is the increase in $\dot{V}O_2$ above pre-exercise values at any time, t; $\Delta\dot{V}O_2(ss)$ is the difference between the pre-exercise and steady state $\dot{V}O_2$; and τ is the time constant (the time it takes to reach 63% [1 - 1/e • 100%] of the rest to steady state value). The time constant, τ characterizes the equation and is determined by iterative fitting programs (Lamarra, 1982). The Phase 2 response represents the combined effects of increases in cardiac output and widening of the $(a-\bar{v})O_2$ difference.

Phase 3 represents the steady state response to a constant power input. The achievement of a steady state for $\dot{V}O_2$ is, in fact, dependent on the relative power performed by the subject. For exercise intensity below the subject's anaerobic threshold (AT), the response characteristics of $\dot{V}O_2$ appear to be linear and first order (i.e., a doubled input of power results in a doubled output of $\dot{V}O_2$ and the time constant is independent of the work rate input). But if work is performed above the subject's AT, then $\dot{V}O_2$ may take longer to achieve a steady state. At sufficiently high work rates, a steady state for $\dot{V}O_2$ is not achieved (Casaburi, Storer, Ben-Dov, & Wasserman, 1987; Figure 3.11). The complexity of these responses for above-the-AT work rates has been the topic of much speculation, the most likely possibility being the additional O_2 requirement for metabolizing excess lactate concentrations that accompany work rate above the AT.

Dynamic $\dot{V}O_2$ Responses in Healthy Children

What has been learned about the growth of the O_2 transport system using the above approach? Cooper, Berry, Lamarra, and Wasserman (1985) hypothesized that the time constant for $\dot{V}O_2$ at the onset of exercise should be independent of body size or age during childhood. The reasoning was as follows: Gas exchange measured at the mouth represents the organism's response to events

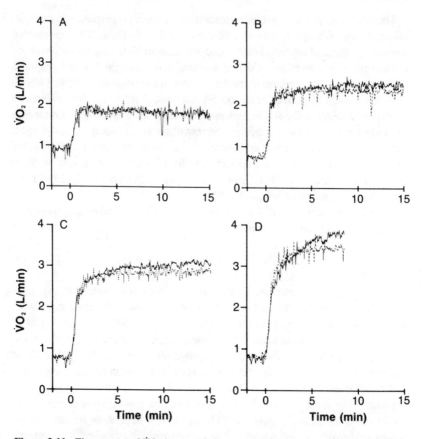

Figure 3.11 Time course of $\dot{V}O_2$ in response to constant power before (solid line) and after (dashed line) endurance training: A, below the subject's anaerobic threshold; B, C, and D, at progressively higher work rates. *Note*. From "Effect of Endurance Training on Possible Determinants of $\dot{V}O_2$ During Heavy Exercise" by R. Casaburi, T.W. Storer, I. Ben-Dov, and K. Wasserman, 1987, *Journal of Applied Physiology, 62*, p. 200. Copyright 1987 by The American Physiological Society. Reprinted by Permission.

occurring at the cellular level. Because these requirements are the same in adults and children (viz., biological similarity), then the response of the whole organism should reflect this similarity. To test this hypothesis, an experiment was done in which transitions between rest and constant work-rate exercise (75% of the subject's AT) were analyzed in 10 younger children (aged 7-9 years) and 10 teenagers (aged 15-18 years). The results of this study are summarized in Figure 3.10. As can be seen, no apparent differences in the characteristics of either Phase 1 or Phase 2 responses could be identified between the younger children and the teenagers.

It is important to note that the constancy of the $\dot{V}O_2$ response occurred despite the fact that other cardiorespiratory frequencies were different in the younger children. Heart rate, for example, is known to be faster in younger children (as it is in smaller compared to larger animals). In the transitions observed in our laboratory, the younger subjects went from generally higher heart rates at rest to generally higher rates during exercise. Interestingly enough, the response time required for the heart rate to achieve a new steady state was slower (expressed as a half-time) in the younger subjects (Cooper, Berry, et al., 1985). Whether the slower response characteristics for heart rate observed in the children represent growth-related differences in responses, or, alternatively, are characteristics of the heart rate response per se is, as yet, unknown.

The independence of the time constant of $\dot{V}O_2$ on body size or age during growth in children implies that the gas exchange system follows first-order, linear kinetics during the growth process. In our study the work rate was scaled to the exercise capability of the children by using the AT as a physiological signpost in subjects of different sizes. The absolute work rate in the teenagers was much greater than in the younger children, but relative to the body mass, the increase in $\dot{V}O_2$ was the same per kilogram in both the teenagers and the younger children. Thus the different work rate inputs resulted in the same relative $\dot{V}O_2$ output (fulfilling the requirements of linearity).

It appears, then, that as children grow, the O_2 transport system changes in such a way that the temporal relationship between $\dot{V}O_2$ at the mouth and cellular O_2 requirement is controlled. Heart size, circulation time, muscle mitochondria, and so forth must change in concert with this regulation.

Dynamic $\dot{V}O_2$ Responses in Disease

What happens when disease impairs the normal growth of the cardiorespiratory system? Sietsema, Cooper, and Perloff (1986) examined the response characteristics to constant work rate in adult patients suffering from inoperable, cyanotic congenital heart disease. Most of these patients had fixed pulmonary hypertension and, hence, were unable to increase pulmonary blood flow normally. The experiment was designed to examine the transition between rest and 0-watt (i.e., unloaded cycling), because most of these patients were unable to exercise at even light work rates. In fact, walking, which involves lifting body mass, represents a greater work load than does unloaded cycling. The ability to examine cardiorespiratory responses at low work rates is important, because in many children with disabilities or chronic disease, maximal progressive exercise protocol may not be safe or desirable.

As can be seen in Figure 3.12, the patients with severe cyanotic congenital heart disease had dramatically reduced response kinetics for oxygen uptake compared to normal controls at the same relative work rates (data represent superimposed, averaged values of breath-by-breath studies). The patients were unable to match $\dot{V}O_2$ with metabolic demand. At present, little is known about the kinetic gas exchange responses either in normal children or in those with chronic disease states. Interestingly, Sady (1981) and Máček and Vávra (1980) examined response kinetics to very high work rates in children and young adults and found differences between the two groups. Did these differences represent

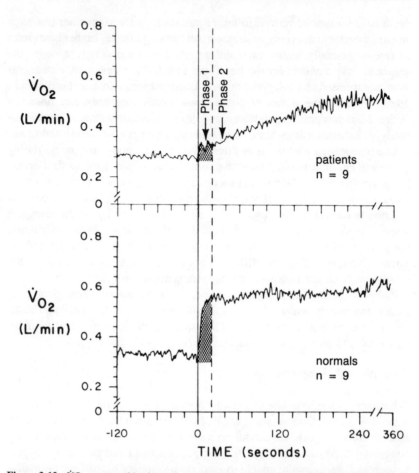

Figure 3.12 $\dot{V}O_2$ response kinetics at the onset of exercise in nine normal subjects and in nine adult patients with cyanotic congenital heart disease. *Note*. From "Dynamics of Oxygen Uptake Exercise in Adults with Cyanotic Congenital Heart Disease" by K.E. Sietsema, D.M. Cooper, and J.F. Perloff, 1986, *Circulation*, **73**, p. 1140. Copyright 1986 by the American Heart Association. Reprinted by permission.

qualitative, growth-related properties in how children and adults respond to high work rates with the accompanying local hypoxia and lactate acidosis? Clearly, more work needs to be done in this potentially important area.

Dynamics of Ventilation in Children

This chapter has focused on the determinants of the growth and development of the O_2 transport system in children. But oxygen uptake is linked both metabolically and structurally to CO_2 production. The maintenance of homeostasis for PCO_2—despite large changes in $\dot{V}CO_2$—is a cardinal feature of respiratory control in both children and adults (Cooper, Kaplan, Baumgarten, & Weiler-

Ravell, 1987). As shown in Figure 3.13, ventilation is linearly related to $\dot{V}CO_2$ during progressive exercise for most of the work rate range. Ventilatory compensation for metabolic acidosis occurs, as shown, at higher work rates and above the respiratory compensation point (RCP). The relationship between ventilation and $\dot{V}CO_2$, specifically, the increase in $\dot{V}_E$ that accompanies an exercise-induced increase in $\dot{V}CO_2$ (see Figure 3.13), is an intensive, qualitative aspect of the cardiorespiratory response in children, in that it represents the ratio of two extensive properties (i.e., ventilation and CO_2 production). Any change in the slope of this relationship ($\Delta\dot{V}_E/\Delta\dot{V}CO_2$) during growth in children is, therefore, likely to reflect maturation of respiratory control in children.

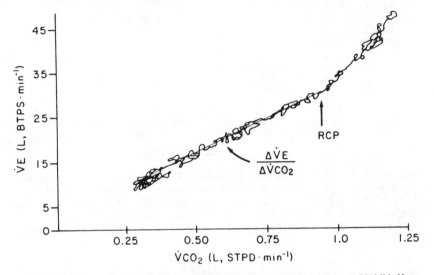

Figure 3.13 $\dot{V}_E$ as a function of $\dot{V}CO_2$ during progressive exercise in an 8-year-old child. *Note.* From "Coupling of Ventilation and CO_2 Production During Exercise in Children" by D.M. Cooper, M.R.Kaplan, L. Baumgarten, and D. Weiler-Ravell, 1987, *Pediatric Research,* **21**, p. 569. Copyright 1987 by Williams & Wilkins. Reprinted by permission.

The slope of the $\dot{V}_E$-$\dot{V}CO_2$ relationship was measured in 128 normal children ranging in age from 6 to 18 years (Cooper et al., 1987). As can be seen in Figure 3.14, there was a small but significant decrease in $\Delta\dot{V}_E/\Delta\dot{V}CO_2$ with increasing age in the children studied. Younger children had to increase ventilation to a greater degree than did older children for a given increase in CO_2 production. An analysis of the alveolar gas equation yields insight into the possible mechanism of these growth-related differences:

$$\dot{V}_E = [863 \cdot P_aCO_2^{-1} \cdot (1 - V_D/V_T)^{-1}] \cdot \dot{V}CO_2 \qquad (10)$$

where $\dot{V}_E$ is ventilation, $\dot{V}CO_2$ is CO_2 production, P_aCO_2 is arterial CO_2 tension, and V_D/V_T is deadspace to tidal volume ratio. As can be seen, the factors affecting the relationship between $\dot{V}_E$ and $\dot{V}CO_2$ will be the P_aCO_2 and the V_D/V_T.

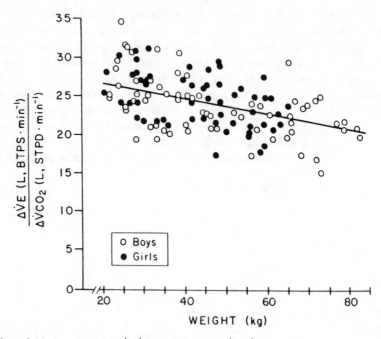

Figure 3.14   The slope of the $\dot{V}_E$-$\dot{V}CO_2$ relationship ($\Delta\dot{V}_E/\Delta\dot{V}CO_2$) in 128 normal children aged 6 to 18 years, showing a small but significant decrease in the relationship with increasing weight in normal children. *Note.* From "Coupling of Ventilation and CO_2 Production During Exercise in Children" by D.M. Cooper, M.R. Kaplan, L. Baumgarten, and D. Weiler-Ravell, 1987, *Pediatric Research,* **21**, p. 569. Copyright 1987 by Williams & Wilkins. Reprinted by permission.

The equation implies that as the regulated level of P_aCO_2 decreases, more ventilation is required for a given increase in $\dot{V}CO_2$. This analysis is consistent with previous work by Godfrey (1974), who found generally lower $PaCO_2$ (arterialized samples) values in younger children (estimated by using arterialized capillary blood) and by observations in this laboratory showing lower end-tidal PCO_2 in younger compared to older children.

We have also analyzed the response kinetics of ventilation and CO_2 production at the onset of exercise in children and teenagers. As shown in Figure 3.15, $\dot{V}CO_2$ and $\dot{V}_E$ lag behind the response of $\dot{V}O_2$ in both children and teenagers, although $\dot{V}CO_2$ and $\dot{V}_E$ were somewhat faster in children than in teenagers. The slowed kinetic response of $\dot{V}CO_2$ is most likely due to the large capacity of the body tissues for CO_2 relative to O_2; thus metabolically produced CO_2 is delayed in its appearance at the mouth by its storage in various tissues. The disparity in the kinetics of $\dot{V}CO_2$ and $\dot{V}O_2$ explains the dip in the respiratory quotient ($\dot{V}CO_2/\dot{V}O_2$) often observed at the onset of exercise. Finally, the figure suggests that $\dot{V}_E$ is coupled with $\dot{V}CO_2$ because the kinetics of these two responses are so similar.

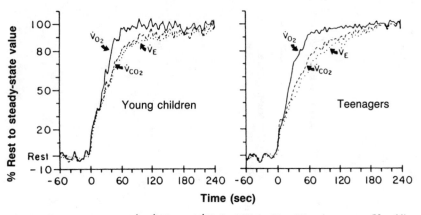

Figure 3.15   The kinetics of $\dot{V}_E$, $\dot{V}CO_2$, and $\dot{V}O_2$ in children ($N = 11$) and teenagers ($N = 11$). *Note.* From "Coupling of Ventilation and CO_2 Production During Exercise in Children" by D.M. Cooper, M.R. Kaplan, L. Baumgarten, and D. Weiler-Ravell, 1987, *Pediatric Research*, **21**, p. 569. Copyright 1987 by Williams & Wilkins. Reprinted by permission.

We were surprised to find that the dynamic response of $\dot{V}CO_2$ and $\dot{V}_E$ were faster in younger compared to older children (Table 3.3). Unlike the response time for $\dot{V}O_2$, the time constants for $\dot{V}_E$ and $\dot{V}CO_2$ appear to be growth related, suggesting that qualitative changes in the control of breathing occur during the growth process. One possible explanation for this observation may be differences in the storage capacity for CO_2 between younger children and adults. Hemoglobin is a major factor for CO_2 transport in the blood, and children have generally lower levels than do adults (Pearson, 1983). Differences in body composition (i.e., proportion of fat and protein) are known to exist between children and young adults (Lohman, Boileau, & Slaughter, 1984), and as the solubility of CO_2 is very large in body fat, the change in body composition may also affect respiratory control in children.

Based on these observations, Springer and Cooper (1987) have begun to examine maturation of respiratory control mechanisms during growth in children. The ventilatory response to progressive exercise was examined in children breathing 15% F_iO_2 and room air. Although a control population of adult subjects invariably increased ventilation when breathing hypoxic gas mixtures, preliminary studies in children have demonstrated a far more varied response, with some subjects demonstrating no response to hypoxia at all. The implications of these studies for maturation of carotid body function during growth in children remain to be elucidated.

Poage, McCann, and Cooper (1987) recently hypothesized that differences in response characteristics of $\dot{V}_E$ and $\dot{V}CO_2$ would be observed when comparing obese to normal children because more metabolically produced CO_2 could be stored in the body tissues in the obese subjects. To test this, ventilatory response kinetics were examined in overweight subjects (children greater than 120%

Table 3.3 Age, Weight, Time Constants for $\dot{V}O_2$, $\dot{V}CO_2$, and $\dot{V}_E$; Preexercise and Mean Exercise $\dot{V}O_2$; and Mean Exercise End-Tidal CO_2 in 11 Younger Children and 11 Teenagers

	Age (yr)	Wt (kg)	$\tau\dot{V}O_2$ (s)	$\tau\dot{V}CO_2$ (s)	$\tau\dot{V}_E$ (s)	Preexercise $\dot{V}O_2$ (L · min^{-1})	Mean exercise $\dot{V}O_2$ (L · min^{-1})	Mean exercise $P_{ET}CO_2$ (mm Hg)
Younger children								
Mean	8.6*	28.4*	26.4	39.9*	41.3*	0.22*	0.68*	39.6*
SD	0.9	3.1	3.2	8.1	12.5	0.04	0.13	1.7
Teenagers								
Mean	17.5	65.9	28.3	50.4	52.4	0.32	1.20	43.5
SD	1.0	10.8	5.6	7.2	9.2	0.06	0.21	2.5

*Significantly differed from teenagers, $p < .05$.

of predicted weight). In preliminary studies, obese children were found to have about 20% longer time constants for $\dot{V}_E$ and $\dot{V}CO_2$ compared to normal subjects. The time constants for $\dot{V}O_2$ did not differ between normal and obese children. The slower ventilatory response times for obese children, despite normal $\dot{V}O_2$ kinetics, implies a reduction in the P_aO_2 at the onset of exercise in these children. Does tissue hypoxia play a role during exercise in these children, rendering activity more uncomfortable? Might this play a role in the lower level of physical activity often observed in obese children?

PHYSICAL ACTIVITY AND CARDIORESPIRATORY GROWTH

The Case of the Kikuyu Women

A number of investigations have attempted to determine the relationship between physical activity and the growth process in children. Most of these studies have focused on the effects in adults of previous activity in competitive sports (Eriksson, Engstrom, & Karlbeyl, 1971; Eriksson, Freychuss, Lundin, & Thoren, 1980), and the results of these studies have not been consistent. But Maloiy and co-workers have recently discovered that habitual activity can profoundly affect the integration of cardiorespiratory and musculoskeletal growth. Their study focused on the Kikuyu and Luo women of Africa who, from early in their childhood, carry loads approximating 70% of their body weight (Maloiy, Heglund, Prager, Cavagna, & Taylor, 1986). Oxygen uptake during treadmill walking was measured in a number of Kikuyu women as they carried loads in their traditional manner (with a band around their foreheads). As can be seen in Figure 3.16, $\dot{V}O_2$ uptake did not increase with increasing loads until the load exceeded approximately 20% of the body weight. In contrast, a group of control women were found to increase $\dot{V}O_2$ directly with increasing loads. The Kikuyu and Luo women may have developed a structural-elastic adaptation to the requirement of carrying heavy loads that tended to minimize energy expenditure. The study points to one area in which physical activity may serve as an important determinant of both metabolic and structural growth.

Relationship Between Mechanical Stress and Growth

Although it is beyond the scope of this discussion to review recent literature concerning lung growth, it is important in this context to point out recent information suggesting the close relationship between the physical process of lung stretching and ultimate lung growth. Using models of unilateral phrenic nerve paralysis, a number of investigators have demonstrated that normal lung growth is inhibited in fetuses and newborn animals without the continuous stretching of lung tissue that normally occurs (Mansell et al., 1986). It has

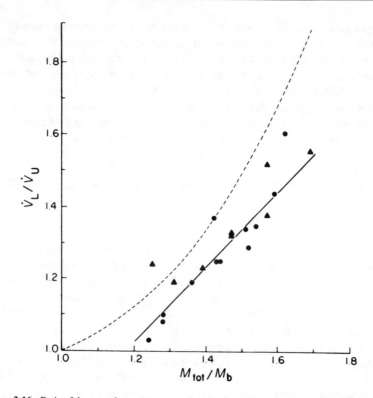

Figure 3.16 Ratio of the rate of oxygen consumption (V) during loaded walking (L) to that during unloaded walking (U) plotted against the ratio of the total mass (Mb + load) to the unloaded mass (M_b) for the Luo and Kikuyu women (solid line) walking at the optimal speed of 3.25 km • h^{-1} compared with the expected relation for army recruits (dashed line). *Note.* From "Energetic Costs of Carrying Loads: Have African Women Discovered an Economic Way?" by G.M.O. Maloiy, N.C. Heglund, L.M. Prager, G.A. Cavagna, and C.R. Taylor, 1986. Reprinted by permission from *Nature*, Vol. 319, Feb. 20-26, p. 669. Copyright © 1986 Macmillan Journals Limited.

been postulated that the release of various growth-stimulating agents may be tied to the stretching of cellular structures. This evidence, tied to the theoretical approaches such as McMahon's elastic similarity, points toward a physiological basis upon which the relationship between physical activity and cardiorespiratory growth may be studied.

DIRECTIONS FOR FUTURE STUDIES

Methodological Problems in Studying Children

In any effort to analyze cardiorespiratory growth in children, attention must be paid to the psychological needs of children in laboratory settings. These concerns, along with the necessity to use noninvasive protocols, has limited the kind of research that can be done in the pediatric age group. Direct measurements of arterial blood, let alone cardiac output or mixed venous blood, are clearly unacceptable. Although in some ways these limitations have been viewed as a hindrance and forced investigators to use animal models in their research efforts, in another sense, these restrictions focused our efforts on studies that can be accomplished in situations approaching real life. Our challenge is to develop increasingly sophisticated and precise tools for noninvasive measurement of gas exchange and O_2 transport in children.

Among the tools currently available for studying children as young as 6 years old is breath-by-breath measurement of gas exchange. I have attempted to demonstrate that, when used with appropriate analytical techniques, these kind of data can yield new insights into the growth process. The high density of breath-by-breath measurements allows accurate assessments of certain dynamic exercise responses from studies of relatively short duration. From a single progressive study, one can evaluate ventilatory function and control ($\Delta\dot{V}_E/\Delta\dot{V}CO_2$), metabolic responses (the anaerobic threshold), and the coupling of respiratory and cardiac function ($\Delta\dot{V}O_2/HR$). Creative uses of different types of forcing functions (e.g., ramp or square-wave protocols with cycle ergometry) can also yield new and nonintuitive information. The time when all pediatric exercise studies relied solely on maximal values has passed, and the standards by which research is judged in our field must begin to reflect new approaches and understanding.

Coupling of Metabolism and Cardiorespiratory Responses During Exercise

We have focused in this chapter on the integration of structure and function during the growth process, with particular emphasis on gas exchange ($\dot{V}CO_2$ and $\dot{V}O_2$). Little attention has been paid to developmental aspects of cellular metabolism during exercise in children. This area has not been well studied because most methodologies for assessing substrate turnover during exercise are invasive and often involve radioactive tracers. However, recently there has been much renewed interest in the use of stable (i.e., nonradioactive) isotopes for physiological research. These isotopes are measured by gas chromatography mass spectrometry, or isotope ratio mass spectrometry. This advance may well benefit pediatric investigators (Wolfe, 1984).

In our own laboratory, for example, we are using the stable isotope of carbon, ^{13}C, to examine the dynamics of the body's bicarbonate compartment at rest and during exercise. This is important because all metabolically produced CO_2 must traverse this compartment in its passage from muscle to atmosphere (N.B., CO_2 is in equilibrium with HCO_3^-). The size and kinetics of this pool critically affect respiratory control, as noted above, and therefore also influence gas exchange in response to exercise, disease, and other stresses. The dynamics of the CO_2-bicarbonate pool are quite likely to change during normal growth and during disease because both hemoglobin levels and body composition changes are a function of growth. Irving, Wong, Shulman, Smith, and Klein (1983) used stable isotopes ^{13}C-bicarbonate to characterize the dynamics of the pool CO_2 in resting subjects, and in preliminary studies, Barstow, Cooper, Sobel, and Epstein (1988) examined CO_2 kinetics during exercise. An interesting feature of the Barstow et al. study is the possibility of using the labeled bicarbonate as a noninvasive method of assessing CO_2 production and, therefore, energy expenditure under field conditions.

In another project, Barstow, Cooper, Epstein, and Wasserman (in press) demonstrated that the mix of metabolic fuel utilization can be estimated simply by measuring the changes in naturally occurring stable isotopes [13]CO_2 in the exhaled breath. This type of analysis must be used with proper attention to the level of exercise (e.g., above or below the anaerobic threshold) as well as to the somewhat complicated dynamics of the CO_2 compartment. However, we believe that these techniques will facilitate new insight into developmental aspects of substrate metabolism.

CONCLUSION

This chapter attempts to develop theoretical and experimental approaches useful for modeling cardiorespiratory growth in children. One can use past efforts of comparative physiologists and theories of biological similarity, but the data suggest that the process of growth in children is a unique case of the relationship between size and function in biology; it is not governed by the same principles that apply to the relationship between size and function in mature animals of different species.

Although the majority of investigations of O_2 transport in children have focused on extensive properties such as maximal oxygen uptake, recent methodological improvements now allow greater attention to intensive properties such as $\Delta \dot{V}_E / \dot{V}CO_2$. I have demonstrated that studying these properties fosters new insight into qualitative changes in the cardiorespiratory system during growth. Moreover, the intensive properties of the organism reflect the control and regulation of the growth process itself. I hope that this approach can be used to understand the biologic basis of physical activity during growth in children.

REFERENCES

Asmussen, E., & Heeboll-Nielsen, K. (1955). A dimensional analysis of physical performance and growth in boys. *Journal of Applied Physiology, 7*, 593-603.

Åstrand, P.O. (1952). *Experimental studies of physical working capacity in relation to sex and age*. Copenhagen: Muskgaard.

Bar-Or, O. (1983). *Pediatric sports medicine for the practitioner*. New York: Springer-Verlag.

Barstow, T., Cooper, D.M., Epstein, S., & Wasserman, K. (in press). Changes in breath $^{13}CO_2/^{12}CO_2$ consequent to exercise and hypoxia. *Journal of Applied Physiology*.

Barstow, T., Cooper, D.M., Sobel, E., & Epstein, S. (1988). Estimation of CO_2 stores by tracer dilution and CO_2 kinetics (Abstract). *FASEBJ.* **2**, A306.

Beaver, W.L., Lamarra, L., & Wasserman, K. (1981). Breath-by-breath measurement of true alveolar gas exchange. *Journal of Applied Physiology*, **51**, 1662-1675.

Casaburi, R., Storer, T.W., Ben-Dov, I., & Wasserman, K. (1987). Effect of endurance training on possible determinants of $\dot{V}O_2$ during heavy exercise. *Journal of Applied Physiology*, **62**, 199-207.

Cooper, D.M., Berry, C., Lamarra, N., & Wasserman, K. (1985). Kinetics of oxygen uptake at the onset of exercise as a function of growth in children. *Journal of Applied Physiology*, **59**, 211-217.

Cooper, D.M., Hyman, C.B., Weiler-Ravell, D., Noble, N.A., Agness, C.L., & Wasserman, K. (1985). Gas exchange during exercise in children with thalassemia major and Diamond-Blackfan anemia. *Pediatric Research*, **19**, 1215-1219.

Cooper, D.M., Kaplan, M.R., Baumgarten, L., & Weiler-Ravell, D. (1987). Coupling of ventilation and CO_2 production during exercise in children. *Pediatric Research*, **21**, 568-572.

Cooper, D.M., Mellins, R.B., & Mansell, A.L. (1981). Changes in distribution of ventilation with lung growth. *Journal of Applied Physiology: Respiratory, Environmental, and Exercise Physiology*, **51**, 699-705.

Cooper, D.M., Weiler-Ravell, D., Whipp, B.J., & Wasserman, K. (1984a). Aerobic parameters of exercise as a function to body size during growth in children. *Journal of Applied Physiology: Respiratory, Environmental, and Exercise Physiology*, **56**, 628-634.

Cooper, D.M., Weiler-Ravell, D., Whipp, B.J., & Wasserman, K. (1984b). Oxygen uptake and heart rate during exercise as a function of growth in children. *Pediatric Research*, **18**, 845-851.

Cunningham, D.A., Paterson, D.H., & Blimkie, C.J.R. (1984). The development of the cardiorespiratory system with growth and physical activity. In R.A. Boileau (Ed.), *Advances in pediatric sports sciences* (pp. 85-116). Champaign, IL: Human Kinetics.

Davies, C.T.M., Barnes, C., & Godfrey, S. (1972). Body composition and maximal exercise performance in children. *Human Biology, 44*, 195-214.

Eriksson, B.O., Engstrom, I., & Karlbeyl, P. (1971). Physiologic analysis of former girl swimmers. *Acta Paediatrica Scandinavica, 217*, 68-72.

Eriksson, B.O., Freychuss, U., Lundin, A., & Thoren, C.A.R. (1980). Effect of physical training in former female top athletes in swimming. In K. Berg & B.O. Eriksson (Eds.), *Children and exercise* (Vol. 9, pp. 116-127). Baltimore: University Park Press.

Feldman, H.A., & McMahon, T.A. (1983). The 3/4 mass exponent for energy metabolism is not a statistical artifact. *Respiratory Physiology, 52*, 149-163.

Godfrey, S. (1974). *Exercise testing in children.* London: W.B. Saunders.

Gould, S.J. (1966). Allometry and size in ontogeny and physiology. *Biological Reviews of the Cambridge Philosophical Society, 41*, 587-640.

Gray, B.F. (1981). On the surface law and basal metabolic rate. *Journal of Theoretical Biology, 93*, 757-767.

Gunther, B. (1975). Dimensional analysis and theory of biological similarity. *Physiological Reviews, 55*, 659-699.

Heusner, A.A. (1982a). Energy metabolism and body size: 1. Is the 0.75 mass exponent of Kleiber's equation a statistical artifact? *Respiration Physiology, 48*, 1-12.

Heusner, A.A. (1982b). Energy metabolism and body size: 2. Dimensional analysis and energetic non-similarity. *Respiration Physiology, 48*, 13-25.

Heusner, A.A. (1983). Body size, energy metabolism, and the lungs. *Journal of Applied Physiology, 54*, 867-873.

Hill, A.V. (1950). The dimensions of animals and their muscular dynamics. *Science Progress, 38*, 208-230.

Irving, C.S., Wong, W.W., Shulman, R.J., Smith, E.O., & Klein, P.D. (1983). [^{13}C]bicarbonate kinetics in humans: Intra- vs. interindividual variations. *Journal of Applied Physiology, 245*, R190-R202.

Kleiber, M. (1975). *The fire of life.* New York: Robert E. Krieger.

Lamarra, N. (1982). *Ventilatory control, cardiac output, and gas-exchange dynamics during exercise transients in man.* Unpublished doctoral dissertation, University of California, Los Angeles.

Lohman, T.G., Boileau, R.A., & Slaughter, M.H. (1984). Body composition in children and youth. In R.A. Boileau (Ed.). *Advances in pediatric sports sciences* (pp. 29-58). Champaign, IL: Human Kinetics.

Máček, M., & Vávra, J. (1980). The adjustment of oxygen uptake at the onset of exercise: A comparison between pre-pubertal boys and young adults. *International Journal of Sports Medicine, 1*, 70-72.

Maloiy, G.M.O., Heglund, N.C., Prager, L.M., Cavagna, G.A., & Taylor, C.R. (1986). Energetic costs of carrying loads: Have African women discovered an economic way? *Nature,* **319,** 668-669.

Mansell, A.L., Rojas, J.V., Sillos, E.M., Stolar, C.J., Collins, M.H., & Rozovski, S.J. (1986). Diaphragmatic activity is a determinant of postnatal lung growth. *Journal of Applied Physiology,* **61,** 1098-1103.

McMahon, T.A. (1973). Size and shape in biology. *Science,* **179,** 1201-1204.

McMahon, T.A. (1984). *Muscles, reflexes, and locomotion.* Princeton: Princeton University Press.

Pearson, H.A. (1983). Diseases of the blood. In R.E. Behrman & E.C. Vaughn (Eds.), *Textbook of pediatrics* (pp. 1204-1257). Philadelphia: W.B. Saunders.

Poage, J., McCann, E.R., & Cooper, D.M. (1987). Ventilatory response to exercise in obese children (Abstract). *American Review of Respiratory Disease,* **135,** A23.

Rosen, R. (1983). Role of similarity principles in data extrapolation. *American Journal of Physiology,* **244,** R591-R599.

Sady, S.P. (1981). Transient oxygen uptake and heart rate responses at the onset of relative endurance exercise in pre-pubertal boys and men. *International Journal of Sports Medicine,* **2,** 240-244.

Schmidt-Nielsen, K. (1972). *How animals work.* Cambridge: Cambridge University Press.

Sietsema, K.E., Cooper, D.M., & Perloff, J.F. (1986). Dynamics of oxygen uptake exercise in adults with cyanotic congenital heart disease. *Circulation,* **73,** 1137-1144.

Springer, C., & Cooper, D.M. (1987). Ventilatory responsiveness to hypoxia during exercise in children and adults (Abstract). *American Review of Respiratory Disease,* **135,** A23.

Taylor, C.R., Maloiy, G.M.O., Weibel, E.R., Langman, V.A., Kamau, J.M.Z., Seeherman, H.J., & Heglund, N.C. (1981). Design of the mammalian respiratory system: 3. Scaling maximum aerobic capacity to body mass: Wild and domestic mammals. *Respiration Physiology,* **44,** 25-38.

Taylor, C.R., & Weibel, E.R. (1981). Design of the mammalian respiratory system: 1. Problems and strategy. *Respiration Physiology,* **44,** 1-10.

Toufexis, A. (1987, January 26). Getting "F" for flabby: U.S. youth comes up short on endurance, strength, and flexibility. *Time,* p. 64.

Von Dobeln, W., Åstrand, I., & Bergstrom, A. (1967). An analysis of age and other factors related to maximal oxygen uptake. *Journal of Applied Physiology,* **22,** 934-938.

Wasserman, K., Hansen, J.E., Sue, D.Y., & Whipp, B.J. (1987). *The principles of exercise testing and interpretation.* Philadelphia: Lea and Febiger.

Wasserman, K., Whipp, B.J., & Davis, J.A. (1981). Respiratory physiology of exercise: Metabolism, gas exchange, and ventilatory control. In J.G. Widdicombe (Ed.), *Respiratory physiology* (Vol. 3, pp. 180-211). Baltimore: University Park Press.

Weibel, E.R. (1984). *The pathway for oxygen. Structure and function in the mammalian respiratory system.* Cambridge: Harvard University Press.

Weibel, E.R., Taylor, C.R., Gehr, P., Hoppeler, H., Mathieu, O., & Maloiy, G.M.O. (1981). Design of the mammalian respiratory system: 9. Functional and structural limits for oxygen flow. *Respiration Physiology, 44*, 151-164.

Whipp, B.J., & Ward, S.A. (1982). Cardiopulmonary coupling during exercise. *Journal of Experimental Biology, 100*, 175-193.

Wilkie, D.R. (1977). Metabolism and body size. In T.J. Pedley (Ed.), *Scale effects in animal locomotion* (pp. 23-26). London: Academic Press.

Wolfe, R.R. (1984). *Tracers in metabolic research.* New York: Alan R. Liss.

Zeltner, T.B., & Burri, P.H. (1987). The postnatal development and growth of the human lung: 2. Morphology. *Respiration Physiology, 67*, 269-282.

Zeltner, T.B., Caduff, J.H., Gehr, P., Pfenninger, J., & Burri, P.H. (1987). The postnatal development and growth of the human lung: 1. Morphometry. *Respiration Physiology, 67*, 247-267.

4

Weight Training in Prepubertal Children: Physiologic Benefit and Potential Damage

Arthur Weltman
University of Virginia

Although increasing muscular strength through weight training is well documented in adults (Atha, 1981), there is controversy regarding the physiologic benefits versus the potential dangers when strength training regimens are applied to prepubertal children.

The American Academy of Pediatrics (1983) has developed an information guide for the pediatrician regarding weight training and weight lifting. In this document *weight training* is defined as "a method of conditioning that involves repetitive action (e.g., biceps curl, shoulder shrug) against submaximum resistance" (p. 157). Submaximum resistance is individualized; it is the amount of weight or resistance that can be taken through the full range of motion for three to four consecutive repetitions. *Weight lifting* is defined as "a sport in which an individual attempts to lift his or her maximum amount of weight" (p. 157). The American Academy of Pediatrics provides the following recommendations regarding weight training and weight lifting:

1. "Weight training utilizes repetitive exercises with weights less than maximum and, when used appropriately, is helpful to athletes in virtually all sports. Weight training, because of the benefits and lower potential for injury, is a reasonably safe technique that, when supervised, can be endorsed for youths" (p. 160).

2. "Prepubertal boys (pubic hair stage 1 or 2) do not significantly improve strength or increase muscle mass in a weight training program because of insufficient circulating androgens" (p. 160).

3. "Maximal benefits are obtained from appropriate weight training in the postpubertal athlete, and minimal benefits are obtained from weight training in the prepubertal athlete" (p. 161).

4. "Weight lifting is a competitive sport with a high injury rate that should not be practiced by the preadolescent" (p. 161).

In contrast, the National Strength and Conditioning Association (1985) has indicated the following:

1. Prepubescent children demonstrate gains in muscular strength as a result of strength training.

2. Because it has been documented that appropriate strengthening of muscle and other tissue can decrease the rate and severity of certain types of sport injuries in adults, and because prepubescent children can increase muscular strength as a result of strength training, it seems logical that similar benefits would occur in the prepubertal population.

3. Psychological benefits, such as improved self-esteem and body image, occur as a result of strength training.

4. Strength training improves motor performance in prepubertal children.

However, at the time of the development and publication of the American Academy of Pediatrics and the National Strength and Conditioning recommendations, little research was available regarding the safety and effectiveness of strength training in prepubertal children. To date, few data exist regarding this issue. The remainder of this chapter reviews available data and provides suggestions for future research.

METHODOLOGICAL CONSIDERATIONS IN
STRENGTH TESTING OF PREPUBESCENT CHILDREN

To accurately measure changes in muscular strength as a result of strength training, it is important to know that strength can be assessed reliably. Furthermore, because the development of muscular strength in children is related to age, body size, previous levels of physical activity, and the various phases of growth (Alexander & Molnar, 1973; Gilliam, Villanacci, Freedson, & Sady, 1979; Molnar & Alexander, 1973, 1974; Tabin, Gregg, & Bonci, 1985; Weltman et al., 1988), it is important, for the purposes of designing exercise training and rehabilitation programs and research designs, to have normative data on the muscular strength in children who differ in maturation levels.

Although limited data regarding the reliability of measuring strength exist for children (Alexander & Molnar, 1973; Gilliam et al., 1979; Molnar & Alexander, 1973, 1974; Tabin et al., 1985; Weltman et al., 1988), normative data for prepubertal boys and girls have not been reported. The lack of such normative data is most likely associated with difficulties in testing large enough samples of young children.

Molnar and Alexander (1973) measured concentric isokinetic strength (Cybex exerciser-dynamometer) for flexion and extension motions at the knee and elbow joints at a velocity of 5 cycles $\cdot$ min^{-1} in 21 girls and 25 boys between the ages of 7 and 15 years. Reliability of strength measurements was determined using a test-retest model and chi-square analysis. Results indicated that no significant differences existed between test and retest strength scores. The authors also reported that strength correlated highly with age, height, and weight ranging from $r = .80$ to $r = .92$. When strength was compared between gender and across age groups the following patterns were observed:

1. Boys were stronger than girls at all ages for all motions.

2. Muscular strength was greater on the dominant side.

3. The strength of the lower extremities was greater than that of the upper extremities, and extension resulted in greater strength than flexion.

4. Strength increased with age, with the greatest increases occurring at the lower extremities and the extensor muscle groups compared to the upper extremities and flexor muscle groups.

Although this study has historical significance in that it showed that strength can be measured reliably in children, it was limited by its small sample size. This resulted in only 1 to 3 subjects in each age group for girls and 0 to 5 subjects in each age group for boys.

Alexander and Molnar (1973) presented similar data on 70 boys and girls between the ages of 7 and 15 and subsequently (Molnar & Alexander, 1974) on 500 normal boys and girls. The authors did not establish norms for muscular strength because they believed that, for such a purpose, data were needed on at least 2,000 boys and girls.

Gilliam et al. (1979) examined differences in isokinetic torque-generating capabilities of young children at the knee and elbow joints for flexion and extension at two speeds (30° and 120° • s^{-1}). The ability to generate torque was examined against age, height, body weight, and gender. Twenty-eight boys and 28 girls were evaluated by means of a Cybex II (Lumex, Inc.) dynamometer. Table 4.1 shows the mean torque for knee and elbow flexion and extension movements at 30° • s^{-1} and 120° • s^{-1}. The means were adjusted (ANCOVA) by sex and corrected for differences that existed in age, height, and body weight.

As can be seen, extension motions resulted in greater torque than flexion motions, and slower speeds resulted in greater torque than faster speeds. When the data were corrected for height, no significant differences were observed between boys and girls for knee torque values. However, boys exhibited significantly greater torque during elbow extension at 120° • s^{-1}. When the effect of body weight on torque-generating capabilities of boys and girls was partialed out, sex differences were observed for knee flexion and extension (girls, 10% less) at 120° • s^{-1}.

Gilliam et al. (1979) also examined the relationship between torque and age, height, and weight. Their data revealed that 45% to 86% of the variability in torque could be explained by differences in age, height, and weight, with correlations higher at the knee joint than the elbow joint. Multiple correlations between collective age, height, and weight and strength did not increase the observed relationships.

Tabin et al. (1985) compared differences in torque-generating capabilities at the knee joint (Cybex dynamometer) in active, healthy males ($N = 30$) and females ($N = 30$). Half of the subjects were prepubescent and half were postpubescent. A nonrandom sample of athletic children was used. Subjects were tested for knee flexion and extension at 60° • s^{-1} and for ankle plantar flexion and dorsiflexion at 30° • s^{-1}. The authors reported their strength scores as torque/lean body weight. However, body composition was measured using anthropometric procedures developed for adults (Sloan, 1967; Sloan, Burt, & Blyth, 1962) and applied to the children of this study. As Lohman, Boileau, and Slaughter (1984) pointed out, the application of adult procedures for estimation of body composition parameters in children may not be appropriate. However, with this limitation in mind, it was shown that few differences existed between boys and girls for quadriceps torque expressed as a function of lean body weight. When Tabin et al. (1985) examined strength ratios, they observed that hamstring strength was approximately 60% of the quadriceps strength. These findings are consistent with several reports (Gilliam et al.,

Table 4.1 Covariate Analyses and Adjusted Mean Scores (± SE) for Knee and Elbow Flexion and Extension Torque (Newton Meters) Values at 30° · s⁻¹ and 120° · s⁻¹ (N = 28 Boys and 28 Girls)

| | | Knee | | | | Elbow | | | |
| | | $30° \cdot s^{-1}$ | | $120° \cdot s^{-1}$ | | $30° \cdot s^{-1}$ | | $120° \cdot s^{-1}$ | |
	Sex	Flexion	Extension	Flexion	Extension	Flexion	Extension	Flexion	Extension
Age[a]	M	22.79 (0.99)	38.57 (1.90)	20.35 (0.83)	27.65 (1.20)	7.00 (0.38)	9.51 (0.47)	6.34 (0.34)	8.33 (0.37)
	F	23.52 (0.94)	39.75 (1.86)	20.05 (0.78)	27.21 (1.14)	6.34 (0.36)	9.07 (0.44)	5.46 (0.32)	7.67 (0.35)
Height[a]	M	24.04 (1.11)	40.27 (2.32)	21.46 (0.93)	28.76 (1.34)	7.37[c] (1.12)	9.81 (0.48)	6.64[c] (0.33)	8.70[b] (0.39)
	F	23.00 (1.00)	38.87 (2.09)	19.62 (0.85)	26.55 (1.21)	6.19 (0.35)	8.92 (1.17)	5.31 (0.30)	7.45 (0.35)
Weight[a]	M	24.11 (0.92)	40.71 (1.90)	21.53[b] (0.83)	29.12[b] (1.10)	7.37[c] (0.35)	9.96 (1.17)	6.56[c] (0.28)	8.70 (0.35)
	F	22.64 (0.85)	38.2 (1.76)	19.32 (0.76)	26.10 (1.01)	6.19 (0.32)	8.85 (0.41)	5.31 (0.30)	7.37 (0.32)

Note. From "Isokinetic Torque in Boys and Girls Ages 7-13: Effect of Age, Height, and Weight" by T.B. Gilliam, J.F. Villanacci, P.S. Freedson, and S. Sady, 1979, *Research Quarterly,* **50**(4), pp. 559-609. Copyright 1979. Reprinted by permission of the American Alliance for Health, Physical Education, Recreation and Dance, 1900 Association Drive, Reston, VA 22091.

[a]All covariates were statistically significant ($p < .05$). [b]Significant sex differences ($p < .05$). [c]Unadjusted means are presented because the slopes between the sexes were unequal ($p < .05$).

1979; Weltman et al., 1988). The ratios for the ankle were different; dorsiflexors produced only 30% of the strength produced by plantar flexors.

To assess whether psychological factors affect the measurement of strength, Molnar, Alexander, and Gutfeld (1979) examined the reliability of quantitative strength measurements (Cybex II) in children with normal intelligence and children with mild mental retardation. Torque was measured during flexion and extension at the elbow and knee joints and during shoulder and hip flexion, extension, and abduction. The study examined (a) intratest variability, (b) intertest variability, and (c) intertester variability. The mean values were consistent for intratest and intertest reliability (a reflection of psychological factors that might affect performance). Intratest variability ranged from 5.4% to 5.9% in the nonretarded population and from 4.9% to 6.2% in the retarded children ($p > .05$). Intertest variability ranged from 7.9% to 9.8% ($p > .05$). Similar results were found for intertester variability: Mean differences of the maximal scores of all muscles combined ranged from 9.0% to 9.7% ($p > .05$). Molnar et al. (1979) concluded that the isokinetic technique of measuring strength is a simple, easily applicable, and reliable method for measuring muscular strength in children with normal intelligence or with a mild degree of mental retardation.

Although most of the research on isokinetic strength measurement in children has used the Cybex dynamometer, Weltman et al. (1988) evaluated the measurement of isokinetic strength in 29 prepubertal boys using a Kin Com isokinetic dynamometer (Chattex, Inc., Chattanooga, TN). Concentric isokinetic strength was evaluated for both the dominant and the nondominant side at the knee, shoulder, and elbow joints. Flexion and extension motions at speeds of $30° \cdot s^{-1}$ and $90° \cdot s^{-1}$ were examined. Because the Kin Com isokinetic dynamometer is designed for adults, modification of the equipment was required to test the boys. Extra support was required behind the seated boy for knee extension, and standing support was required for elbow flexion and extension. This was necessary to raise the boys to an appropriate height and for stabilization to prevent substitution by the paravertebral muscles during elbow flexion and the abdominal muscles during elbow extension. Modification of adult testing equipment is a major methodological constraint when trying to collect reliable strength data in children.

Table 4.2 shows the mean work output (joules) per repetition at the knee, shoulder, and elbow joints found by Weltman et al. (1988). At the knee joint, extension at $30° \cdot s^{-1}$ resulted in 56% greater work output than felxion at $30° \cdot s^{-1}$, and extension at $90° \cdot s^{-1}$ resulted in 52% greater work output than flexion at $90° \cdot s^{-1}$. At $30° \cdot s^{-1}$, the hamstrings-to-quadriceps strength ratios were 63.6% (dominant side) and 64.6% (nondominant side). At $90° \cdot s^{-1}$, the relative hamstring strength was 64.2% for the dominant side and 67.5% for the nondominant side. Mean work output during flexion at $90° \cdot s^{-1}$ was approximately 15% lower than mean work output during flexion at $30° \cdot s^{-1}$. Similar results were found for extension; mean work output at $90° \cdot s^{-1}$ was

Table 4.2 Mean Work Output (Joules) at the Knee, Shoulder, and Elbow Joints for Flexion and Extension Motions at 30° · s^{-1} and 90° · s^{-1}, N = 29

Motion	Dominant (M ± SD)	Nondominant (M ± SD)	Correlation[a] coefficient
		Knee	
Flexion			
30° · s^{-1}	19.6 ± 5.5	21.4 ± 6.8	.81
90° · s^{-1}	16.5 ± 4.9	18.3 ± 6.2	.73
Extension			
30° · s^{-1}	30.8 ± 13.0	33.1 ± 14.1	.91
90° · s^{-1}	25.7 ± 11.5	27.1 ± 11.7	.90
		Shoulder	
Flexion			
30° · s^{-1}	15.9 ± 4.4	15.2 ± 5.1	.62
90° · s^{-1}	13.2 ± 4.0	12.6 ± 4.7	.39
Extension			
30° · s^{-1}	23.6 ± 6.9	23.9 ± 8.4	.87
90° · s^{-1}	20.1 ± 6.3	20.3 ± 6.8	.87
		Elbow	
Flexion			
30° · s^{-1}	10.4 ± 3.7	10.7 ± 3.4	.72
90° · s^{-1}	9.3 ± 3.9	9.7 ± 3.0	.78
Extension			
30° · s^{-1}	11.5 ± 3.2	10.7 ± 3.9	.79
90° · s^{-1}	10.3 ± 3.4	8.7 ± 3.3	.73

Note. From "Measurement of Isokinetic Strength in Pre-Pubertal Males" by A. Weltman, S. Tippett, C. Janney, K. Strand, C. Rians, B.R. Cahill, and F.I. Katch, 1988, *Journal of Orthopaedic and Sports Physical Therapy, 9*(10), p. 347. Copyright 1988 by the Journal of Orthopaedic and Sports Physical Therapy. Reprinted by permission.

[a]$r \geqslant .36$ for $p < .05$.

approximately 81-83% of mean work output at 30° · s^{-1}. Similar findings were observed at the shoulder and elbow joints, with extension resulting in greater mean work output than flexion and the slow speed resulting in greater work output than the faster speed (Table 4.2).

Although test-retest reliability was not measured, an estimate was obtained by comparing the outputs measured between the dominant and nondominant sides for each motion (Table 4.2). The correlations ranged from $r = .72$ to $r = .91$ for all motions, with the exception of shoulder flexion, where $r < .70$. Reliability was also estimated by examining torque scores throughout the entire range of motion between the dominant and the nondominant sides. With the exception of the two shoulder flexion motions, the correlations between torque for all motions (between the dominant and the nondominant sides) were in the range of $r = .60$ to $r = .90$. The correlations for shoulder flexion were lower than those observed for other motions, suggesting that individual inconsistencies in torque for this motion may not yield reliable data for prepubertal boys.

The above results suggest that prepubertal boys, if properly positioned, can be evaluated for concentric isokinetic muscular strength for knee flexion and extension, elbow flexion and extension, and shoulder extension motions at speeds of $30° \cdot s^{-1}$ and $90° \cdot s^{-1}$. Results observed for shoulder flexion movements were not as reproducible as the other motions evaluated. The data reveal that evaluation of shoulder flexion strength may have limited value in prepubertal children. It was consistently observed that prepubertal children relied on extensive muscle substitution to complete the shoulder flexion motion. Isolating the anterior deltoid was difficult in these young boys, resulting in probable substitution from the long head of the biceps and extension of the trunk and contralateral trunk flexors. This may help explain the lower reliability for this motion.

Weltman et al. (1988) also found that prepubertal boys developed similar patterns of strength throughout the range of motion as compared to adults. As observed with adults, prepubertal boys developed greater torque during extension compared to flexion and at slower compared to faster isokinetic speeds. In addition, the torque curves observed for prepubertal boys (Figures 4.1-4.3) are similar to adult torque curves (Knapik, Wright, Nawdsley, & Brun, 1983), in that peak torque levels were developed during the initial phases of the range of motion.

In summary, these data support the assumption that prepubertal children can have isokinetic muscular strength assessed in a reliable and reproducible manner, provided that they are properly positioned and that the available isokinetic dynamometers are' adjusted (i.e., padded) appropriately. However, it should be noted that the data reviewed in the previous section were collected on children 6 years of age or older. The ability to measure strength reliability in younger subjects has not been addressed. Finally, other methodological constraints in strength assessment must be addressed when conducting longitudinal studies. These include changes in growth, maturation, and learning, as well as ability of the habitual physical activity of children. These constraints demonstrate the need for appropriate control groups when collecting longitudinal data in children.

CHANGES ASSOCIATED WITH STRENGTH TRAINING IN PREPUBERTAL CHILDREN

Relatively few studies have examined the effectiveness and safety of strength training in prepubertal children. This lack of data may be related to conten-

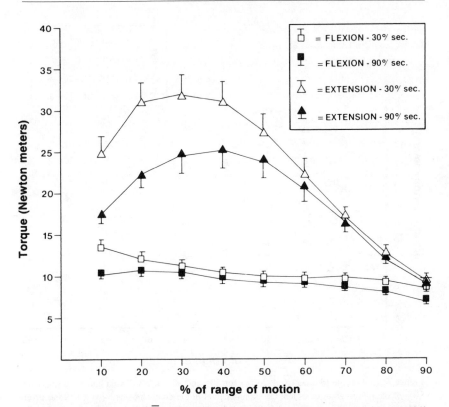

Figure 4.1   Average torques ($\overline{X} \pm$ SEM) FOR 30° and 90° • s⁻¹ flexion and extension over 90 % of the full range of motion at the knee joint of the dominant side, $N = 29$. *Note*. From "Measurement of Isokinetic Strength in Pre-Pubertal Males" by A. Weltman, S. Tippett, C. Janney, K. Strand, C. Rians, B.R. Cahill, and F.I. Katch, 1988, *Journal of Orthopaedic and Sports Physical Therapy,* 9(10), p. 349. Copyright 1988 by the Journal of Orthopaedic and Sports Physical Therapy. Reprinted by permission.

tions that prepubertal children should not engage in strength training because (a) they lack adequate levels of circulating androgens and therefore are incapable of increasing muscular strength as a result of strength training; (b) those strength gains that might be attainable in prepubertal children would not improve sports performance or reduce the risk of injury in this population; and (c) strength training is dangerous for prepubertal children, resulting in a high risk of injury. The available data do not support these contentions. This section reviews such data regarding the effectiveness of strength training in prepubertal children.

Muscular Strength

One of the first studies that specifically examined the ability of prepubertal boys to strength-train was conducted by Vrijens (1978). He strength-trained two groups of children: a prepubertal group ($N = 16$, mean age = 10 years,

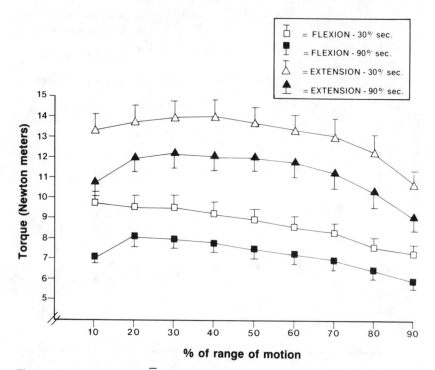

Figure 4.2 Average torques ($\overline{X}$ ± SEM) for 30° and 90° % s^{-1} flexion and extension over 90% of the full range of motion at the shoulder joint of the dominant side, $N = 29$. *Note.* From "Measurement of Isokinetic Strength in Pre-Pubertal Males" by A. Weltman, S. Tippett, C. Janney, K. Strand, C. Rians, B.R. Cahill, and F.I. Katch, 1988, *Journal of Orthopaedic and Sports Physical Therapy,* 9(10), p. 350. Copyright 1988 by the Journal of Orthopaedic and Sports Physical Therapy. Reprinted by permission.

5 months) and an adolescent group ($N = 12$, mean age = 16 years, 8 months). Subjects were trained using isotonic exercises, performed in a circuit of 8 exercises, with 8-12 repetitions per exercise. Subjects trained three times per week for 8 weeks. Subjects were assessed before and after the training period for muscular strength (measured isometrically), muscular hypertrophy (soft-tissue roentegenography), and changes in anthropometric measures.

Changes in isometric strength as a result of isotonic strength training are presented in Table 4.3. For the prepubertal boys no consistent pattern of strength improvement was observed. They improved strength in the abdominal and back muscles with no change in strength in the upper and lower extremities. In contrast, the adolescents improved strength in all muscle groups tested. The improvement in strength in the adolscent group and the lack of improvement in the prepubertal group was confirmed by roentgenographic measurements (Table 4.4). The adolescent group showed a significant increase of muscle mass in the arm and thigh, whereas no changes were noticed in prepubertal boys.

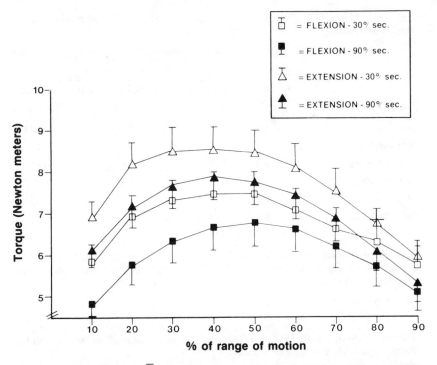

Figure 4.3 Average torques ($\overline{X} \pm$ SEM) for 30° and 90° • s⁻¹ flexion and extension over 90% of the full range of motion at the elbow joint of the dominant side, $N = 29$. *Note*. From "Measurement of Isokinetic Strength in Pre-Pubertal Males" by A. Weltman, S. Tippett, C. Janney, K. Strand, C. Rians, B.R. Cahill, and F.I. Katch, 1988, *Journal of Orthopaedic and Sports Physical Therapy*, **9**(10), p. 350. Copyright 1988 by the Journal of Orthopaedic and Sports Physical Therapy. Reprinted by permission.

Vrijens (1978) concluded that the lack of strength improvement in the prepubertal boys was due to the fact that, before physical maturation, muscle weight takes up a small percentage of body weight in boys and that prior to puberty little change in muscle mass is possible. After sexual maturation, muscular development is enhanced by androgenic hormones, and muscle weight increases to about 40% of body weight. This allows for increased strength as a result of training. Although Vrijens (1978) noted that Grimm and Reade (1967) and Rohmert (1968) reported that strength development can occur in prepubertal children, Vrijens concluded that, in childhood, variations in training responses only occur during growth.

The study by Vrijens (1978) is often cited as part of the rationale for not instituting strength training programs for prepubertal children (American Academy of Pediatrics, 1983; Pfeiffer & Francis, 1986; Weltman et al., 1986), but several methodological problems are associated with that report: (a) no control group was included, (b) subjects completed only one set of repetitions

Table 4.3   Mean Values for Isometric Strength (in Newtons) Before and After 8 Weeks of Training

	Prepubescent (N = 16)			Postpubescent (N = 12)		
	Before	After	Difference	Before	After	Difference
Arm flexors	1.3	1.2	−0.1	2.4	2.8	+0.4**
Arm extensors	1.0	1.1	+0.1	1.6	2.1	+0.5*
Leg extensors	2.2	2.0	−0.2	4.8	2.1	+0.9**
Leg flexors	1.5	1.5	+0.0	2.3	3.0	+0.7***
Abdomen	1.7	2.3	+0.6***	4.4	5.5	+1.1**
Back muscles	5.0	6.8	+1.8***	12.0	13.9	+1.9**

Note. From "Muscle Strength Development in the Pre- and Post-Pubescent Age" by J. Vrijens, 1978, *Medicine Sport*, **11**, pp. 152-158. Copyright 1978 by S. Karger AG, Basel. Adapted by permission.
*$p < .05$. **$p < .02$. ***$p < .01$.

Table 4.4   Mean Values for Cross-Sectional Surface Area (cm²) of Muscle and Fat Before and After 8 Weeks of Training

	Prepubescent (N = 16)			Postpubescent (N = 12)		
	Before	After	Difference	Before	After	Difference
Thigh						
Muscle	101.8	103.0	+1.2	185.7	194.2	+8.5*
Fat	34.8	34.6	−0.2	42.1	37.2	−5.0*
Arm						
Muscle	25.4	26.0	+0.6	43.5	49.7	+6.2**
Fat	13.3	12.9	−0.4	13.2	12.4	−0.8

Note. From "Muscle Strength Development in the Pre- and Post-Pubescent Age" by J. Vrijens, 1978, *Medicine Sport*, **11**, pp. 152-158. Copyright 1978 by S. Karger AG, Basel. Adapted by permission.
*$p < .05$. **$p < .02$.

per exercise station (this may not have resulted in a large enough stimulus to induce changes in strength in prepubertal boys), and (c) subjects trained dynamically and were tested statically (the concept of specificity of training suggests that the strength training and evaluation modes should be similar).

Nielsen, Nielsen, Behrendt Hansen, and Asmussen (1980) also examined training modes in children. They trained 249 girls aged 7-19 for 5 weeks. Subjects were assigned to one of three training groups: isometrics, trained with isometric knee extensions; jumpers, trained using vertical jumps; and runners, trained by sprinting. The girls were evaluated before and after training for isometric strength, vertical jump, and acceleration (10-m sprint). Results indicated that the girls had the largest training effects in the tests for which they were specifically trained. The younger (< 13.5 years of age) and smaller (< 155 cm) girls who trained isometrically had a greater percent improvement in isometric strength than the group as a whole. Nielsen et al. (1980) concluded that the increase in girls' muscle strength with age is partly a result of a dimensional growth in height and weight as well as an age factor (which presumably improves neuromuscular function), but their data also suggest that younger and smaller girls can also gain strength as a result of specific strength training.

Three recent studies further support the effectiveness of appropriate strength training regimens in prepubertal children (Pfeiffer & Francis, 1986; Sewall & Micheli, 1986; Weltman et al., 1986). Sewall and Micheli divided 18 boys and girls aged 10-11 into strength training (8 boys, 2 girls, 9 Tanner Stage I, 1 Tanner Stage II) and control (7 boys, 1 girl, 7 Tanner Stage I, 1 Tanner Stage II) groups. The training group trained 3 days per week for 9 weeks. The training sessions consisted of a flexibility routine followed by a warm-up and strength training. Strength training consisted of three sets of 10 or more repetitions of resistive weight training on the Nautilus thigh press machine, the Cam II chest press machine, and the Cam II row machine. The sets were performed as follows: first set, 10 reps at 50% of 10 repetition maximum (10 RM); second set, 10 reps at 80% 10 RM; and third set, as many reps as possible at 100% 10RM. When subjects were able to complete 12 repetitions at 100% 10 RM, resistance was increased. The children were closely supervised, with one instructor supervising groups of three or four children. After the strength training phase, 9 weeks of detraining was initiated.

Results of Sewall and Micheli (1986; see Table 4.5) revealed that the strength-trained subjects recorded greater strength improvements than the control group, with statistically significant improvements observed for shoulder flexion ($p <.05$). They concluded that strength gains are possible in prepubertal children when children are placed on a proper resistive exercise program. Of the four motions studied, knee extension, shoulder flexion, and shoulder extension showed greater increases in the strength-trained group. Strength was measured isometrically whereas the actual training techniques were performed with dynamic contractions, which, the authors argued, supports the contention that true strength gains were observed rather than neuromuscular adaptations to patterned motion.

Pfeiffer and Francis (1986) compared responses to strength training in 80 male children, adolescents, and adults. Subjects were divided into prepubescent, pubescent, and postpubescent groups and were randomly assigned to

Table 4.5   Percentage Increase in Strength

	Knee extension	Knee flexion	Shoulder flexion	Shoulder extension	Mean
Strength training	30.3	12.6	95.8*	32.9	42.9
Control	12.3	12.1	17.9*	−4.1	9.5

Note. From "Strength Training for Children" by L. Sewall and L.J. Micheli, 1986, *Journal of Pediatric Orthopedics*, **6**, pp. 143-146. Reprinted by permission.

*$p < .05$.

strength training and control groups. The strength of elbow and knee flexors and extensors was assessed bilaterally at $30° • s^{-1}$ and $120° • s^{-1}$ using a Cybex isokinetic dynamometer. Subjects trained 3 days per week for 9 weeks and performed three sets of 10 repetitions (50% 10 RM, 75% 10 RM, 100% 10 RM) of leg extension, leg curl, bench press, and biceps curl. In addition, one set of rowing, shoulder extension, leg press, sit-ups, and butterflies was performed. Subjects strength-trained using Universal Machines and free weights. They were closely supervised with six to eight subjects per exercise leader.

The training group, regardless of maturity level, showed a significant increase in strength in all of the upper extremity motions. Only knee extension increased at the knee joint in the training group compared to the controls. Regardless of pubertal state, the percent change in torque/kilogram body weight was similar in the strength training groups (Figures 4.4 and 4.5). Indeed, in the right limbs, the only significant difference observed among the groups of boys with differing pubertal status was a significantly greater improvement in knee flexion at $30° • s^{-1}$ in the prepubescents compared to the pubescents (Figure 4.5). Similar results were observed among the three pubertal states when the left limbs were examined: All strength training groups showed similar improvements in strength, with the prepubescent group exhibiting significantly greater percentage improvements for elbow flexion and knee extension at $120° • s^{-1}$ compared to the pubescent and postpubescent groups.

The study cited demonstrates that males of differing pubertal status can gain strength as a result of a well-supervised resistive exercise program. The fact that the effects of training were similar across maturity levels further supports the hypothesis that prepubertal children can benefit from a strength training program.

Weltman et al. (1986) examined the effects of hydraulic resistance strength training on 16 prepubertal boys using Hydra-Fitness equipment; 10 prepubertal boys served as controls. Subjects participated in a closely supervised, 3 days/week, 14-week strength training program. Each session was 45 min in

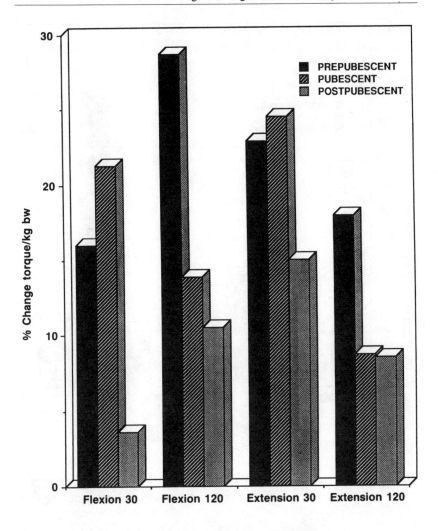

Figure 4.4 Mean strength changes for right elbow flexion and extension of the experimental group according to maturity level. *Note*. From "Effects of Strength Training on Muscle Development in Prepubescent, Pubescent, and Postpubescent Males" by R.D. Pfeiffer and R.S. Francis, 1986, *The Physician and Sportsmedicine*, **14**(9), p. 138. Copyright 1986 by McGraw-Hill. Reprinted by permission of THE PHYSICIAN AND SPORTSMEDICINE, a McGraw-Hill publication.

duration and consisted of 5 to 7 min of warm-up exercises (including stretching), 30 min of strength training, and 5 to 7 min of cool-down exercises (including stretching). Circuit strength training was performed using eight hydraulic resistive machines. The hydraulic resistance devices allowed for

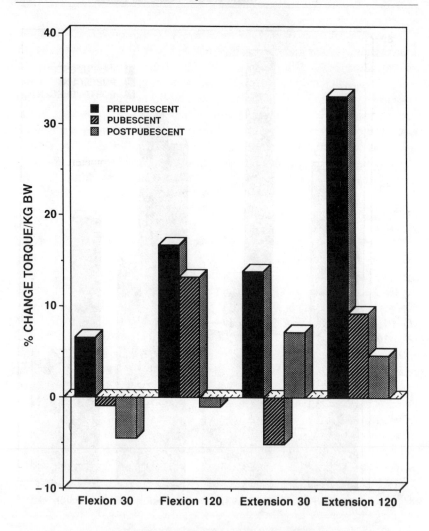

Figure 4.5   Mean strength changes for right knee flexion and extension of the experimental group according to maturity level. *Note.* From "Effects of Strength Training on Muscle Development in Prepubescent, Pubescent, and Postpubescent Males" by R.D. Pfeiffer and R.S. Francis, 1986, *The Physician and Sportsmedicine*, **14**(9), p. 138. Copyright 1986 by McGraw-Hill. Reprinted by permission of THE PHYSICIAN AND SPORTSMEDICINE, a McGraw-Hill publication.

concentric reciprocal movement and included the following: biceps/triceps, bench press, quadriceps/hamstring, shoulder press, abduction/adduction hip, butterfly, forearm conditioner, and jump squat. The equipment needed to be modified (i.e., padded) in order to accommodate the boys.

One circuit consisted of exercise for 30 s with a 30-s rest between stations. Subjects attempted as many repetitions as possible in 30 s. All subjects began training at the lowest of six resistance settings. When 30 or more repetitions, at a given setting, could be performed the subject was allowed to advance the resistance by one setting. Each subject completed three circuits during a strength training session. No strength training activities were allowed outside of the supervised program. Control subjects continued to participate in their organized sport activities and activities of daily living (ADL) during the 14 weeks. Strength was measured using a Kin Com isokinetic dynamometer. Subjects were evaluated for concentric strength at the knee and elbow joints for both flexion and extension at speeds of $30°$ and $90° \cdot s^{-1}$. Average concentric work and average torque at each 10% of the range of motion (ROM) were also measured.

Table 4.6 indicates that the strength training group gained in strength in all eight motions (percent change ranged from $+18.5\%$ to $+36.6\%$). For all but three motions, a significant two-way interaction was present, indicating that the change in mean work for the strength training group was greater than the change in mean work for the control group ($p < .05$). A similar trend was observed for the three motions in which significant two-way interactions were not present.

Weltman et al. (1986) also examined changes in torque scores over the full ROM (Figure 4.6). For knee extension ($30° \cdot s^{-1}$) the training group showed increased torque ranging from $+16.9\%$ (40% ROM) to $+42.2\%$ (80% ROM), whereas the change in torque in the control group ranged from -8.1% (60% ROM) to $+9.9\%$ (10% ROM).

Statistical analysis revealed that a significant two-way interaction (i.e., the improvement in the strength training group was greater [$p < .05$] than the change in the control group) was present over the entire ROM. Similar results were observed for knee extension at $90° \cdot s^{-1}$ and knee flexion at $30°$ and $90° \cdot s^{-1}$. In other words, torque improved in the training group throughout the range of motion; improvements ranged from 13% to 43% depending on motion and percent of ROM. Significant two-way interactions were observed for the entire ROM. Similar results were also observed when the four elbow motions were examined.

The major finding of Weltman et al. (1986) was that a short-term, closely supervised resistance strength training program that used hydraulic exercise devices significantly increased concentric isokinetic strength in prepubertal boys. They suggested that prepubertal boys can increase strength in spite of low levels of androgens (testosterone levels of less than $20 \text{ ng} \cdot dL^{-1}$, dihydroepiandosterone-sulfate [DHEA-S] levels less than $600 \text{ ng} \cdot mL^{-1}$). The improvement in strength was not surprising because muscular hypertrophy is only one of the physiological adaptions that may be responsible for training-induced improvements in neuromuscular power (Coyle et al., 1981). Several

Table 4.6 Changes in Average Isokinetic Concentric Work (in Joules) Per Repetition as a Result of Strength Training in Prepubertal Boys

Movement	ROM	Average concentric work per repetition [M, (SD)]					
		Strength training (N = 16)			Control (N = 10)		
		Pre	Post	% Change	Pre	Post	% Change
Knee							
Flexion 30° · s^{-1}	110°	19.5 (5.4)	24.1 (7.5)	+23.6	21.1 (5.9)	20.9 (5.9)	− 1.0[a, b]
Flexion 90° · s^{-1}	110°	16.2 (3.8)	19.6 (6.3)	+21.0	18.1 (6.4)	17.1 (4.9)	− 5.5[a, b]
Extension 30° · s^{-1}	90°	26.9(10.3)	33.5(12.2)	+24.5	38.5(15.6)	38.4(18.3)	− 0.3[a, b]
Extension 90° · s^{-1}	90°	23.6 (9.1)	28.0(13.1)	+18.6	31.0(14.8)	32.5(17.6)	+ 4.8[a]
Elbow							
Flexion 30° · s^{-1}	90°	11.3 (3.7)	14.6 (5.5)	+29.2	9.6 (4.0)	9.5 (4.1)	− 1.0[a, b]
Flexion 90° · s^{-1}	90°	10.1 (4.0)	13.8 (5.7)	+36.6	8.5 (4.1)	9.0 (3.6)	+ 5.9[a, b]
Extension 30° · s^{-1}	90°	11.5 (3.3)	15.2 (3.6)	+32.1	11.7 (3.7)	13.4 (5.3)	+14.5[a]
Extension 90° · s^{-1}	90°	11.2 (3.2)	13.3 (3.3)	+18.5	9.6 (3.9)	11.0 (4.8)	+14.6[a]

Note. From A. Weltman, C. Janney, C.B. Rians, K. Strand, B. Berg, S. Tippet, J. Wise, B.R. Cahill, and F.I. Katch, "The Effects of Hydraulic Resistance Strength Training in Pre-Pubertal Males," in *Medicine and Science in Sports and Exercise*, **18**(6), pp. 629-638, © by American College of Sports Medicine, 1986. Adapted by permission.

[a]Main effect, post > pre, $p < .05$. [b]Significant two-way interaction, $p < .05$.

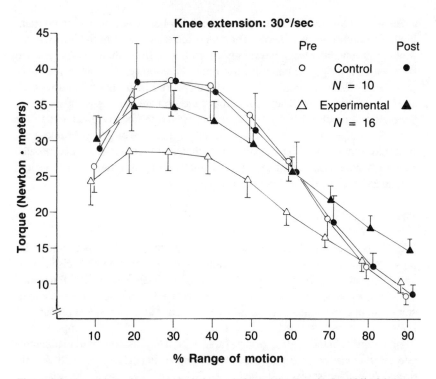

Figure 4.6 Comparison of torque scores before and after training over the first 90% of the range of motion, for knee extension: 30° • s⁻¹. *Note*. From "The Effects of Hydraulic Resistance Strength Training in Pre-Pubertal Males" by A. Weltman, C. Janney, C.B. Rians, K. Strand, B. Berg, S. Tippett, J. Wise, B.R. Cahill, and F.I. Katch, 1986, *Medicine and Science in Sports and Exercise*, **18**(6), 629-638. Copyright 1986 by the American College of Sports Medicine. Adapted by permission.

factors, such as the number of motor units recruited and their synchronization, may also control the development of neuromuscular power. In support of this hypothesis, Hakkinen and Komi (1983) reported that initial increases in strength as a result of strength training can be accounted for by neural factors rather than by muscle hypertrophy. Weltman et al. (1986) suggest that, because muscular strength increased in the absence of changes in circumferences, the increases in strength observed in the prepubertal boys were probably the result of neural adaptations.

Flexibility

One concern about strength training is that flexibility may be compromised as a result of resistive exercises. However, the available data suggest that, as long as stretching and flexibility exercises are included as part of a strength training program, flexibility may actually increase.

Sewall and Micheli (1986) measured flexibility before and after strength training their prepubescent subjects. They reported slight gains in flexibility in the training group after strength training. More importantly, their results revealed that resistive weight training did not reduce flexibility. Similar results were reported by Weltman et al. (1986), who measured flexibility of the low back and hamstring muscles. They reported that the strength training group increased their sit-and-reach score by 8.4%, which was significantly greater than the −1.2% change in sit-and-reach observed in the control group (Table 4.7). It should be noted that both Sewall and Micheli and Weltman et al. incorporated flexibility exercises as part of their strength training programs. This ensured that ROM and flexibility were maintained.

Physical Performance

It could be speculated that motor performance that involves neuromuscular power should be enhanced after strength training. The data of Nielsen et al. and Weltman et al. (1986) support this suggestion. Nielsen et al. (1980) reported that girls, irrespective of age and size, who trained with isometric knee extensions also improved their vertical jump. Weltman et al. reported that prepubertal boys who strength-trained increased vertical jump by 10.4% compared to a 3% decrement in the control group (Table 4.7). They also reported that parents perceived that strength training resulted in improved performance in their childrens' organized sports activities.

Body Composition

Weltman et al. (1986) measured circumferences, skinfolds, and body density before and after their 14-week experimental period. Circumferences were taken at the head, neck, shoulders, chest, waist, umbilicus, buttocks, thighs, knees, calves, ankles, deltoids, biceps flexed, biceps extended, forearms, and wrists. Skinfolds were taken at the chin, chest, scapula, triceps, mid-axillary, waist, suprailiac, abdominal, thigh, knee, and calf sites. Body density was assessed by hydrostatic weighting.

Results indicated that both the control and strength training groups increased in height and weight; the strength training group gained more weight than the controls (Table 4.7). No changes were observed for body density or skinfold measures. For circumferences the only sites that changed significantly were at the shoulder, chest, and average abdomen (increased circumferences in the strength training group). These results differ from previous findings in adults indicating that both men and women can reduce percent body fat and skinfold thickness consequent to short-term strength training (Wilmore, 1974). However, it is difficult to assess the effects of strength training on body composition in prepubertal boys because they are simultaneously involved in the growth and development process while training.

Table 4.7 Changes in $\dot{V}O_2$max and Related Variables as a Result of Strength Training in Prepubertal Boys

Variable	Strength training (N = 16)			Control (N = 10)		
	Pre M (SD)	Post M (SD)	% Change	Pre M (SD)	Post M (SD)	% Change
Sit and reach (cm)	39.2 (6.4)	42.5 (6.2)	+ 8.4	38.5 (3.0)	38.0 (3.8)	− 1.2[a, b]
Vertical jump (cm)	21.1 (4.8)	23.3 (3.4)	+10.4	22.7 (3.9)	22.0 (2.5)	− 3.0[a, b]
Height (cm)	134.0 (7.0)	136.0 (7.1)	+ 1.5	132.5 (9.3)	133.4 (9.0)	+ 0.7[a]
Weight (kg)	29.87 (6.84)	31.50 (7.59)	+ 5.5	27.32 (6.12)	27.91 (5.54)	+ 2.2[a, b]
Body density (g $\cdot$ cm^{-3})	1.060(0.018)	1.056(0.018)	− 0.4	1.052(0.013)	1.056(0.008)	+ 0.4
$\dot{V}O_2$max (L $\cdot$ min^{-1})	1.39 (0.26)	1.66 (0.32)	+19.4	1.48 (0.31)	1.44 (0.26)	− 2.7[a, b]
$\dot{V}O_2$max (mL $\cdot$ kg $\cdot$ min^{-1})	46.79 (3.48)	53.23 (4.61)	+13.8	54.62 (3.12)	51.69 (2.59)	− 5.4[a, b]
Treadmill time (min)	15.0 (1.9)	17.1 (1.9)	+14.0	17.0 (1.5)	16.9 (1.7)	− 0.5[a, b]
Respiratory exchange ratio	1.00 (0.05)	1.03 (0.05)	+ 3.0	1.01 (0.05)	1.02 (0.04)	+ 1.0
Maximal heart rate	197.8 (5.2)	199.9 (5.7)	+ 1.1	200.5 (9.0)	196.9 (7.2)	− 1.8

Note. From A. Weltman, C. Janney, C.B. Rians, K. Strand, B. Berg, S. Tippet, J. Wise, B.R. Cahill, and F.I. Katch, "The Effects of Hydraulic Resistance Strength Training in Pre-Pubertal Males" in *Medicine and Science in Sports and Exercise*, **18**(6), pp. 629-638, © by American College of Sports Medicine, 1986. Adapted by permission.

[a]Main effect post > pre, $p < .05$. [b]Significant two-way interaction, $p < .05$.

Maximal Oxygen Consumption

Weltman et al. (1986) also evaluated changes in maximal oxygen consumption ($\dot{V}O_2$max) consequent to strength training in prepubertal boys (Table 4.7). $\dot{V}O_2$max increased in the strength training group ($+19.4\%$ and $+13.8\%$ when expressed in L • min^{-1} and mL • kg^{-1} • min^{-1}, respectively). The control group showed decreases in $\dot{V}O_2$max of -2.7% (L • min^{-1}) and -5.4% (mL • kg^{-1} • min^{-1}; significant two-way interaction, $p < .05$). Similar results were observed for total treadmill time. No significant differences were observed between groups or before or after training for respiratory exchange ratio and maximal heart rate. These results differ from recent findings regarding strength training and $\dot{V}O_2$max changes in adults (Hurley et al., 1984). Although 16 weeks of high-intensity variable resistance Nautilus strength training (using the manufacturer's recommendations) increased strength in adult males, $\dot{V}O_2$max was not affected by Nautilus training. Perhaps the increase in $\dot{V}O_2$max observed by Weltman et al. (1986) was related to the reciprocal concentric nature of the hydraulic resistance training devices and the volume of exercise performed in a given training session. In support of the hypothesis described, Katch, Freedson, and Jones (1985) reported that the MET level and calorie expenditure of hydraulic resistance exercise were considerably higher than values compared for exercise using free weights, Nautilus, or Universal Gym equipment. This increased energy expenditure may help to explain the increase observed in $\dot{V}O_2$max in the study by Weltman et al. Similar results for young boys who were involved in a hydraulic resistance strength training program were recently reported by Doucherty, Wenger, and Collis (1987). Both relative and absolute $\dot{V}O_2$max increased independent of whether subjects trained in a high-velocity/low-resistance mode or a low-velocity/high-resistance mode. In addition, as Gettman and Pollock (1981) pointed out, improvement in $\dot{V}O_2$max as a result of circuit weight training depends on the amount of work performed. The fact that three sets of up to 30 repetitions per set were performed may also have contributed to the increase in $\dot{V}O_2$max observed by Weltman et al. (1986).

Health-Related Variables

Serum Lipid Levels. Weltman, Janney, Rians, Strand, and Katch (1987) examined the effects of hydraulic resistance strength training on changes in serum lipid levels of prepubertal boys. Their results indicated that boys who strength-trained reduced serum cholesterol by 15.7% (5.09 mmol • L^{-1} pretraining, 4.30 mmol • L-1 posttraining; $p < .05$) and total/HDL-C by 17.9% (3.52 pretraining, 2.89 posttraining; $p < .05$). The reduction observed in serum cholesterol of 0.80 mmol • L^{-1} in the strength training group was considerably higher than the 0.26-mmol • L^{-1} average decrease usually seen in serum cholesterol as a result of exercise (Tran, Weltman, Glass, & Mood, 1983), but was similar to previously reported findings regarding strength training in adult males and females (Goldberg, Elliot, Schultz, & Kloster, 1984). It should be noted that the initial serum cholesterol level of 5.09 mmol • L^{-1} for the strength training group was considerably (p < .05) higher than the initial serum cholesterol level of 4.14 mmol • L^{-1} observed in the control group, and was also elevated above the recommended cholesterol levels of 4.65 mmol • L^{-1} for young children. As Tran et al. (1983) pointed out, elevated initial levels of serum cholesterol are more easily reduced by exercise training than are lower initial levels of serum cholesterol. The elevated initial levels of serum cholesterol observed by Weltman et al. (1987) may, in part, explain the favorable reduction in serum cholesterol and total/HDL-C observed. Furthermore, the hydraulic resistance exercise used in this study also resulted in an increase in V̇O₂max. As such, the reduction in total cholesterol cannot be ascribed entirely to strength training alone.

Hypertension.   Although no data are available regarding the effects of strength training on hypertension in prepubertal children, Hagberg et al. (1984) have examined the effects of weight training on blood pressure and hemodynamic variables in hypertensive adolescents. They studied six adolescents with persistent essential hypertension. They reported that initial endurance training significantly lowered blood pressure at rest (systolic blood pressure decreased from 143 to 130 mm Hg [p < 05], diastolic pressure decreased from 80 to 77 mm Hg). Subsequent weight training did not elevate blood pressure. Although the V̇O₂max increases observed as a result of endurance training decreased significantly during strength training, systolic and diastolic blood pressure remained lower after strength training (126 mm Hg and 73 mm Hg, respectively). In one subject who did not participate in endurance training, strength training alone resulted in similar decreases in blood pressure. Cessation of training resulted in elevation of blood pressure to levels that were not different from those measured prior to training. Hagberg et al. concluded that strenuous weight training can maintain the reduction in blood pressure elicited by endurance exercise training and in some cases may elicit a reduction in blood pressure without prior endurance training. They further concluded that in hypertensive adolescents, whose blood pressure is not as elevated as in older hypertensive populations, weight training may be useful in controlling the hypertensive state.

Other Disease States.   Little information exists regarding strength training and pediatric diseases in which exercise is used as a therapy. For example, Bar-Or (1983) suggests that in progressive muscular dystrophy abnormal changes in the affected muscle fibers will continue, but physical conditioning can improve the function of the residual, healthy muscle fibers. Strength training may be an effective form of therapy in prepubertal children with certain neuromuscular diseases, provided they are able to perform this activity (Vignos & Watkins, 1966).

SAFETY OF STRENGTH TRAINING
IN PREPUBERTAL CHILDREN

A major concern regarding strength training for prepubertal children is the possibility of increased risk of injury to the musculoskeletal system. Micheli (1984) has suggested that the growing bones and joints of a child are more susceptible to certain types of injury than those of an adult. In particular, Micheli stated that the growth plate and articular surface of the child are more susceptible to shear and impact injury and that the presence of growth cartilage at the tendon insertions increases the chance of avulsion from the bone.

Existing evidence indicates that the preadolescent athlete has a lower risk of injury than high school or college athletes, even when participating in organized contact sports (Micheli, 1984), but some data indicate that Olympic lifting movements and weight training can result in injuries in adolescents (Brady, Cahill, & Bodnar, 1982; Jesse, 1977). However, most of the injuries observed usually occur in poorly supervised settings; when maximal weight is used through extremes of joint motion, which the musculature of the young child may not be strong enough to control; or when ballistic movements, such as those seen in Olympic weight lifting, are used.

In weight training settings that employ proper supervision, training-related injuries in children are very low (Rians et al., 1987; Sewall & Micheli, 1986; Weltman et al., 1986). Sewall and Micheli (1986) did not observe any injuries as a result of strength training in their prepubertal boys. Rians et al. (1987) examined the safety aspects of the strength training performed by the prepubertal boys of the Weltman et al. (1986) study using the following methods:

1. Injury surveillance was conducted. Those injuries occurring during strength training were noted separately from those occurring during sports and activities of daily living. Injuries were defined as those complaints that resulted in an inability to complete the circuit or complete absence from a session.

2. Subclinical deleterious effects of strength training on the musculoskeletal system were investigated using biphasic musculoskeletal scintigraphy (bone, epiphyses, and muscle) as well as measurement of serum creatine phosphokinase, a muscle enzyme released during muscle necrosis. Scintigraphy was performed using a pediatric dose (Young's rule) of technitium 99 m pyrophosphate with imaging by a long field of view camera of the appendicular skeleton at 5 min (muscle phase) and 2 hr (skeletal phase). Scintigraphy was done on 8 of 10 controls and 17 of 18 experimental subjects.

Results of the safety analysis were as follows: Injury surveillance revealed one strength-training-related injury, whereas six injuries occurred in sports and activities of daily living. The strength training injury occurred during the shoulder press and diagnosis of shoulder strain was made. The boy's symptoms resolved with 1 week of rest from the shoulder press, while complet the other stations. No other strength-training-related injuries were found, thou multiple complaints occurred. In every other case, the musculoskeletal co plaint was resolved by correction of technique. Many such corrections were required, indicating the high level of supervision necessary to avoid incorrect technique and potential injury.

Injuries occurring during activities of daily living included a gastrocnemius strain, a clavicle fracture, a contusion of the knee, and a contused iliac crest. Sports injuries included a contusion of the clavicle and a contusion of the first metatarsal, in both cases caused by contact in hockey. Absences from strength training as a result of these injuries numbered 47 of a total 756 subject sessions, compared to the 3 absences caused by the one strength training injury. This was a 16-fold difference.

Creatine phosphokinase levels were not elevated in either group either before or after the strengthening program. Scintigraphy revealed no evidence of muscle damage in any subject. Comparison of the epiphyseal plates before and after strength training and between control and experimental groups revealed no differences. Two experimental subjects had abnormal scans after strength training in anatomic locations that were scintigraphically normal prior to training. In one subject the left tibia was normal prior to training and abnormal after training. This subject complained of being hit in the left tibia with a hockey puck in the day or two preceding the postscintigraphic evaluation. In two other ice hockey players who showed similar abnormalities before strength training, the abnormalities resolved in spite of strength training. Therefore, the abnormality of the tibia after strength training in the one subject was judged to be the result of trauma incurred during sports activity.

The second scintigraphic abnormality after strength training involved increased activity in the distal ulna and radial epiphysis. When the scintigraphic abnormality was discovered, it was revealed that the subject had a history of repeated falls on the outstretched hand during basketball competition. His tenderness had resolved 1 month after stopping basketball, in spite of continuing strength training, suggesting that strength training had little or nothing to do with this abnormal scan. Rians et al. (1987) concluded that a closely supervised, primarily concentric strength training program for prepubescent males results in a low musculoskeletal injury rate. However, as Rians et al. and others (Sewall & Micheli, 1986) have emphasized, only carefully supervised programs are associated with low risk of injury. It is generally agreed upon that unsupervised strength training programs may result in increased risk of serious injury in prepubertal children.

CONCLUSION

In conclusion, the available data indicate that (a) isokinetic strength can be reliably and reproducibly measured in prepubertal children provided the equipment is modified appropriately; and (b) in the short term (i.e., less than 14 weeks), prepubertal children can adapt to a strength training program with increases in strength and improvements in other physiological parameters without undue risk of injury. However, if a young child is to participate in a strength training program it is important to follow these guidelines:

1. A careful preparticipation evaluation should be performed to rule out contraindications to any specific exercise.

2. The program must be closely supervised by knowledgeable, trained individuals.

3. Emphasis in the strength training program should be placed on proper form.

4. Lifting maximal weight as well as performing ballistic movements should be avoided until skeletal maturity is attained.

CHALLENGES FOR FUTURE RESEARCH

The responses to strength training in young children present an open and challenging field for future research. There are numerous unanswered questions regarding the maturation process and the effectiveness and safety of strength training. The following are some suggested topics for further study.

- What are the effects of long-term strength training in young children?
- Is there a gender difference in the ability of young children to strength-train?
- Is there a difference in the rate of strength development based upon pubertal state?
- Does strength training in young children affect bone mineral content?
- Are there differences in effectiveness and injury rates between modalities of strength training that use primarily concentric contractions and those that use both concentric and eccentric exercises?

REFERENCES

Alexander, J., & Molnar, G.E. (1973). Muscular strength in children: Preliminary report on objective standards. *Archives of Physical Medicine and Rehabilitation,* **54**, 424-427.

American Academy of Pediatrics (1983). Weight training and weight lifting: Information for the pediatrician. *The Physician and Sportsmedicine,* **11**, 157-161.

Atha, J. (1981). Strengthening muscle. *Exercise and Sport Science Reviews,* **91**, 1-73.

Bar-Or, O. (1983). *Pediatric sports medicine for the practitioner*. New York: Springer-Verlag.

Brady, T.A., Cahill, B.R., & Bodnar, L. (1982). Weight training-related injuries. *American Journal of Sports Medicine, 10*, 1-5.

Coyle, E.F., Feiring, D.C., Rotkins, T.C., Cote, R.W., III, Robey, F.B., Lee, W., & Wilmore, J.H. (1981). Specificity of power improvements through slow and fast isokinetic training. *Journal of Applied Physiology: Respiratory, Environmental and Exercise Physiology, 51*, 1437-1442.

Doucherty, D., Wenger, H.A., & Collis, M.L. (1987). The effects of resistance training on aerobic and anaerobic power of young boys. *Medicine and Science in Sports and Exercise, 19*, 389-392.

Gettman, L.R., & Pollock, M.L. (1981). Circuit weight training: A critical review of its benefits. *The Physician and Sportsmedicine, 9*, 44-60.

Gilliam, T.B., Villanacci, J.F., Freedson, P.S., & Sady, S. (1979). Isokinetic torque in boys and girls ages 7-13: Effect of age, height and weight. *Research Quarterly, 50*, 559-609.

Goldberg, L., Elliot, D.L., Schultz, R.W., & Kloster, F.E. (1984). Changes in lipid and lipoprotein levels after weight training. *Journal of American Medical Association, 252*, 504-506.

Grimm, D., & Reade, H. (1967). Erfolgreiche Anwendung des kreisbetriebs in einer 3. klasse. *Theorie und Praxis der Körpekultur, 16*, 333-342.

Hagberg, J.M., Ehsani, A.A., Goldring, D., Hernandez, A., Sinacore, D.R., & Holloszy, J.O. (1984). Effect of weight training on blood pressure and hemodynamics in hypertensive adolescents. *Journal of Pediatrics, 104*, 147-151.

Hakkinen, K., & Komi, P.V. (1983). Electromyographic changes during strength training and detraining. *Medicine and Science in Sports and Exercise, 15*, 455-460.

Hurley, B.F., Seals, D.R., Ehsani, A.A., Cartier, L.J., Dalsky, G.P., Hagberg, J.M., & Hollosy, J.O. (1984). Effects of high intensity strength training on cardiovascular function. *Medicine and Science in Sports and Exercise, 16*, 483-488.

Jesse, J.P. (1977). Olympic lifting movements endanger adolescent weight lifters. *The Physician and Sportsmedicine, 9*, 61-67.

Katch, F.I., Freedson, P.S., & Jones, C.A. (1985). Evaluation of acute cardio-respiratory responses to hydraulic resistance exercise. *Medicine and Science in Sports and Exercise, 17*, 168-173.

Knapik, J.J., Wright, J.E., Nawdsley, R.H., & Brun, J. (1983). Isometric, isotonic and isokinetic torque variations in four muscle groups through a range of joint motion. *Physical Therapy, 63*, 938-947.

Lohman, T.G., Boileau, R.A., & Slaughter, M.H. (1984). Body composition in children and youth. *Advances in Pediatric Sport Sciences*, **1**, 29-57.

Micheli, L.J. (1984). Sport injuries in the young athete: Questions and controversies. In L.J. Micheli (Ed.), *Pediatric and adolescent sports medicine* (pp. 1-9). Boston: Little, Brown.

Molnar, G.E., & Alexander, J. (1973). Quantitative muscle testing in children: A pilot study. *Archives of Physical Medicine and Rehabilitation*, **54**, 224-228.

Molnar, G.E., & Alexander, J. (1974). Development of quantitative standards for muscle strength in children. *Archives of Physical Medicine and Rehabilitation*, **55**, 490-493.

Molnar, G.E., Alexander, J., & Gutfeld, N. (1979). Reliability of quantitative strength measurements in children. *Archives of Physical Medicine Rehabilitation*, **60**, 218-221.

National Strength and Conditioning Association (1985). Position paper on prepubescent strength training. *National Strength and Conditioning Association Journal*, **7**, 27-29.

Nielsen, B., Nielsen, K., Behrendt Hansen, M., & Asmussen, A. (1980). Training of function muscular strength in girls 7-19 years old. In K. Berg & B.K. Erikson (Eds.), *Children and exercise*, (Vol. 9, pp. 69-78). Baltimore: University Park Press.

Pfeiffer, R.D., & Francis, R.S. (1986). Effects of strength training on muscle development in prepubescent, pubescent, and postpubescent males. *The Physician and Sportsmedicine*, **14**(9), 134-143.

Rians, C.B., Weltman, A., Cahill, B.R., Janney, C.A., Tippett, S.R., & Katch, F.I. (1987). Strength training for prepubescent males: Is it safe? *American Journal of Sports Medicine*, **15**, 483-489.

Rohmert, W. (1968). Rechts-Links-Vergleich bei sometrischem Armmuskeltraining mit verschiedenem Trairingsreiz bei achtjahrigen Kindren. *Internationale Zeitschrift für Angewandte Physiologie*, **26**, 363-393.

Sewall, L., & Micheli, L.J. (1986). Strength training for children. *Journal of Pediatric Orthopedics*, **6**, 143-146.

Sloan, A.W. (1967). Estimation of body fat in young men. *Journal of Applied Physiology*, **23**, 311-315.

Sloan, A.W., Burt, J.J., & Blyth, D.S. (1962). Estimation of body fat in young women. *Journal of Applied Physiology*, **17**, 967-970.

Tabin, G.C., Gregg, J.R., & Bonci, T. (1985). Predictive leg strength values in immediately prepubescent and postpubescent athletes. *American Journal of Sports Medicine*, **13**, 387-389.

Tran, Z.V., Weltman, A., Glass, G., & Mood, D. (1983). The effects of exercise on blood lipids and lipoproteins: A meta-analysis of studies. *Medicine and Science in Sports and Exercise,* **15**, 393-402.

Vignos, P.J., & Watkins, M.P. (1966). The effect of exercise in muscular dystrophy. *Journal of the American Medical Association,* **197**, 843-848.

Vrijens, J. (1978). Muscle strength development in the pre- and post-pubescent age. *Medicine Sport,* **11**, 152-158.

Weltman, A., Janney, C., Rians, C.B., Strand, K., Berg, B., Tippett, S., Wise, J., Cahill, B.R., & Katch, F.I. (1986). The effects of hydraulic resistance strength training in pre-pubertal males. *Medicine and Science in Sports and Exercise,* **18**, 629-638.

Weltman, A., Janney, C., Rians, C.B., Strand, K., & Katch, F.I. (1987). The effects of hydraulic-resistance strength training on serum lipid levels in prepubertal boys. *American Journal of Diseases in Children,* **141**, 777-780.

Weltman, A., Tippett, S., Janney, C., Strand, K., Rians, C., Cahill, B.R., & Katch, F.I. (1988). Measurement of isokinetic strength in pre-pubertal males. *Journal of Orthopaedic and Sports Physical Therapy,* **9**, 345-351.

Wilmore, J.H. (1974). Alterations in strength, body composition and anthropometric measurements consequent to a 10-week weight training program. *Medicine and Science in Sports,* **6**, 133-138.

5

The Use of the Anaerobic Threshold in Pediatric Exercise Testing

Tony M. Reybrouck
Univeristy of Leuven, Belgium

During an incremental exercise test a critical exercise intensity can be identified at which a disproportionate increase is found for pulmonary ventilation ($\dot{V}_E$) and lactate relative to oxygen uptake ($\dot{V}O_2$; Figure 5.1). Because of the coincidence of the changes in $\dot{V}_E$ and lactate under normal conditions, this exercise intensity has been designated as the *anaerobic threshold* (AT) by Wasserman, Whipp, Koyal, and Beaver (1973) and has been considered to be an indirect estimate for the onset of metabolic acidosis during graded exercise.

In adults, AT correlates well with other indexes of aerobic function such as $\dot{V}O_2$max and maximal endurance performance (Reybrouck, Ghesquiere, Cattaert, Fagard, & Amery, 1983; Reybrouck, Ghesquiere, Weymans, & Amery, 1986; Wasserman, 1984).

Children have more difficulty than adults in performing a true maximal effort and reaching a plateau of $\dot{V}O_2$ with increasing exercise intensity, as required

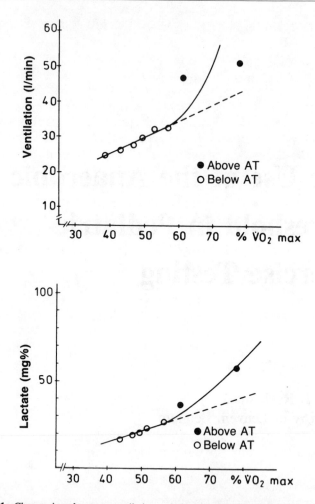

Figure 5.1 Changes in pulmonary ventilation and plasma lactate during graded exercise below and above the anaerobic threshold (AT) in a representative subject. *Note.* From "Ventilatory Thresholds During Short- and Long-Term Exercise" by T. Reybrouck, J. Ghesquiere, A. Cattaert, R. Fagard, and A. Amery, 1983, *Journal of Applied Physiology, 55,* p. 1698. Copyright 1983 by The American Physiological Society. Adapted by permission.

to have an objective and reliable assessment of $\dot{V}O_2$max (Cunningham, Van Waterschoot, Paterson, Lefcoe, & Sangal, 1977). Therefore, the use of AT to determine cardiorespiratory endurance capacity is advantageous in the pediatric age group, as it can be determined during a submaximal exercise test, which obviates the need of maximal exercise testing. (For a more detailed discussion on the historical background and development of the concept of anaerobic threshold, see Jones & Ehrsam, 1982; Margaria, 1979; Stremel, 1984; and Wasserman, Hansen, Sue, & Whipp, 1987.)

CONTROVERSIES IN THE ANAEROBIC THRESHOLD CONCEPT

Despite the many studies that reported a simultaneous change in lactate and onset of hyperventilation (for references see Jones & Ehrsam, 1982; McLellan, 1985; Wasserman et al., 1973), a number of investigators disagree on the causal relationship between metabolic acidosis and the onset of hyperventilation (Brooks, 1985; Gladden, 1984; Jones & Ehrsam, 1982). In experimental studies (e.g., after glycogen depletion) a divergence between the lactate threshold and the ventilatory threshold could be shown (Hughes, Turner, & Brooks, 1982). Therefore, a cause-and-effect relationship is not always warranted. Because the AT, both in adults (Reybrouck et al., 1983) and children (Reybrouck, Weymans, Ghesquiere, Van Gerven, & Stijns, 1982), correlates well with other indexes of aerobic function such as $\dot{V}O_2max$ and maximal endurance performance, it should be considered as an index of cardiorespiratory endurance performance capacity, whether the plasma lactate response has been shown to coincide with pulmonary ventilation or not.

To avoid misunderstanding or discussions about cause and effect, it may be more appropriate to use the term *ventilatory threshold*, which does not imply a link with anaerobic metabolism. However, because the concept has originally been defined as anaerobic threshold (Wasserman et al., 1973) and because this term is still most widely used (Tavazzi & di Prampero, 1986), it is used in this chapter.

ANAEROBIC THRESHOLD IN CHILDREN

Application of Lactate and Ventilatory Threshold Concept

Although a ventilatory breaking point or lactate breaking point during graded exercise was first described in adults, the same phenomenon can be detected in children (Figure 5.2). In exercise studies on 99 children, aged 6 to 14 years, Máček and Vávra (1985) found that the threshold for a disproportionate increase in $\dot{V}_E$ was correlated with the threshold for plasma lactate increase. As with observations in adults, in healthy children, aged 9 to 15 years, a concomitant disproportionate increase of lactate concentration and a nonlinear increase in $\dot{V}_E$ during graded exercise can also be deduced from published experimental data (Eriksson, 1972; Eriksson & Koch, 1973; Gadhoke & Jones, 1973; Máček & Vávra, 1969). Also, the use of a fixed blood lactate level of 4 mmol • L^{-1} (Gaisl & Wiesspeiner, 1986), or a delta base deficit of 4.5 mmol • L^{-1} (Gaisl & Buchberger, 1982), has been used to identify the AT in children and adolescents.

In experimental studies on young children, we could already detect a ventilatory threshold during treadmill exercise in kindergarten children. The AT in

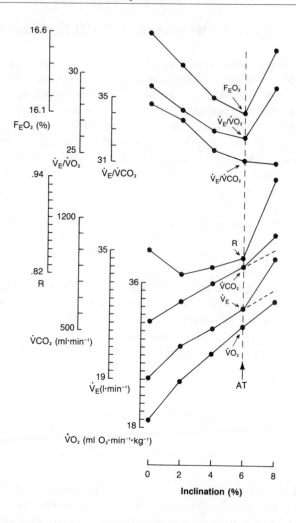

Figure 5.2 Changes of respiratory variables below and above the anaerobic threshold (AT) during graded exercise on a treadmill in a representative child. *Note.* From "Ventilatory Threshold in Healthy Children: Age and Sex Differences," by T. Reybrouck, M. Weymans, H. Stijns, J. Knops, and L. Van der Hauwaert, 1985, *European Journal of Applied Physiology,* **54,** p. 279. Copyright 1985 by Dr. Wolf Isselhard. Reprinted by permission.

kindergarten children correlated well with another parameter of aerobic function: the PWC170, the physical work capacity at a heart rate of 170 beats • min^{-1} (Figure 5.3). Similarly, Cooper, Weiler-Ravell, Whipp, and Wasserman (1984) identified a ventilatory (anaerobic) threshold in young children from the age of 6 years onwards. (Note: Both PWC170 and AT may be expressed in mL O_2 • min^{-1}.)

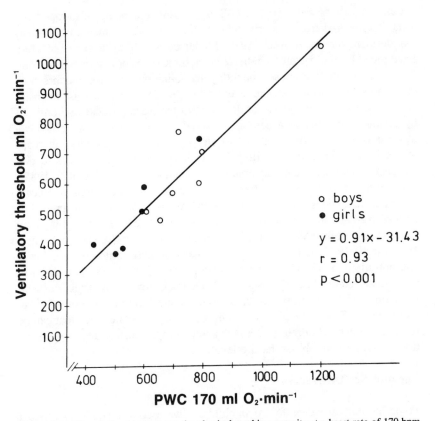

Figure 5.3   The relationship between the physical working capacity at a heart rate of 170 bpm (PWC170) and the ventilatory (anaerobic) threshold, both expressed in mL O_2 • min⁻¹, in kindergarten children. *Note*. From "Ventilatory Threshold During Treadmill Exercise in Kindergarten Children" by T. Reybrouck, M. Weymans, J. Ghesquiere, D. Van Gerven, and H. Stijns, 1982, *European Journal of Applied Physiology, 50*, p. 81. Copyright 1982 by Dr. Wolf Isselhard. Reprinted by permission.

Criteria for Detection of Anaerobic Threshold

Currently used criteria to detect the AT, using breath-by-breath gas exchange are (a) an increase of the ventilatory equivalent for oxygen uptake ($\dot{V}_E/\dot{V}O_2$) without a concomitant increase in the ventilatory equivalent for CO_2 output ($\dot{V}_E/\dot{V}CO_2$) and (b) an increase in end-tidal PO_2 without an increase in end-tidal PCO_2 (Wasserman, 1984; Whipp, Davis, Torres, & Wasserman, 1981). However, when using average values over a whole minute for these ventilatory equivalents, researchers can apply the same criteria (Figure 5.2; Caiozzo et al., 1982; Davis, 1985; Davis, Vodak, Wilmore, Vodak, & Kurtz, 1976; Kremser & Rajfer, 1986; Reybrouck et al., 1983; Wasserman & Whipp, 1975).

Following the initial reports on AT, other researchers also developed criteria that differed from the original definition of AT. German physiologists (Kinderman, Simon, & Keul, 1979; Mader et al., 1976) proposed to use a fixed blood level of lactate to indicate the aerobic or anaerobic threshold. Kinderman et al. (1979) proposed the following definitions: The aerobic threshold corresponds to a plasma lactate level of 2 mmol • L^{-1} (this exercise intensity corresponds to a first significant deviation of the plasma lactate and onset of hyperventilation); and the anaerobic threshold, defined at a plasma lactate level of 4 mmol • L^{-1}, corresponds to the steep part of the exponential increase of the lactate concentration. Both lactate levels enable researchers to discriminate performance capacity among different individuals (McLellan, 1985).

A limitation for the use of a fixed blood lactate level in children to indicate the AT is that it does not represent the same relative exercise intensity in children as in adults. In children, the maximal blood lactate levels are significantly lower than in adults (Åstrand, 1952; Cunningham et al., 1977; Davies, Barnes, & Godfrey, 1972; Eriksson, 1972), perhaps because children have lower concentrations of the glycolytic enzyme phosphofructokinase compared to values obtained in adults (Eriksson, 1972; Gollnick, Armstrong, Saubert, Piehl, & Saltin, 1972). Therefore, a fixed blood lactate level of 4 mmol • L^{-1}, to indicate the AT, may be close to the maximal blood lactate value that can be reached in young children, whereas in adults it represents a much lower fraction of the maximal blood lactate level.

Age and Sex Differences

To define normal values for At in children, we used a treadmill to conduct exercise testing on 257 healthy children (140 boys and 117 girls) spanning the ages of 6 to 18 years (Reybrouck, Weymans, Stijns, Knops, & Van der Hauwaert, 1985). Contrary to the mild increase of $\dot{V}O_2$max, expressed as mL • min^{-1} • kg^{-1} in the 6- to 16-year-old boys, the AT, also expressed as mL • min^{-1} • kg^{-1}, was significantly lower in the 15- to 18-year-olds than in the 6- to 12-year-olds (Figure 5.4). In girls, no significant age-related change in $\dot{V}O_2$max was observed. For the AT, a more complex curve was found in girls. It was highest in the youngest age group, decreased around 7 years, and increased again between 10 and 12 years. It was also lowest in the oldest girls (15 to 16 years, Figure 5.4).

In comparing the gender groups, we found that the AT was reached at a significantly lower $\dot{V}O_2$ in the girls than in boys of the same age. This is in agreement with earlier observations of Máček and Vávra (1971), who found that anaerobiosis starts at a lower exercise intensity in girls than in boys of the same age.

A major finding is the significant decrease of the AT in growing children when expressed as a percent of $\dot{V}O_2$max (Figure 5.4). The same has been reported by Cooper et al. (1984), using the cycle ergometer. This results from the interaction of changes in $\dot{V}O_2$max (mL • min^{-1} • kg^{-1}) and AT

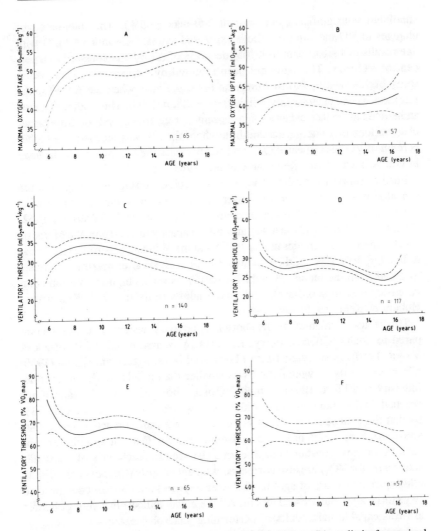

Figure 5.4 Normal range, expressed by a polynome with 95% confidence limits for maximal oxygen uptake in boys (A) and girls (B), ventilatory anaerobic threshold in boys (C) and girls (D), and ventilatory anaerobic threshold (expressed as a percent of $\dot{V}O_2$max in boys (E) and girls (F). Ages ranged from 5 to 18 years. *Note.* From "Ventilatory Anaerobic Threshold in Healthy Children: Age and Sex Differences" by T. Reybrouck, M. Weymans, H. Stijns, J. Knops, and L. Van der Hauwaert, 1985, *European Journal of Applied Physiology,* **54**, p. 280. Copyright 1985 by Dr. Wolf Isselhard. Reprinted by permission.

(mL • min^{-1} • kg^{-1}) with age. In boys, the AT decreases at a rate greater than the rise in $\dot{V}O_2$max (mL • min^{-1} • kg^{-1}) in the 9- to 14-year-olds (-16% for the AT and $+4\%$ for $\dot{V}O_2$max). Therefore it is obvious that AT, when expressed as a percentage of $\dot{V}O_2$max, decreases with age in boys. Similarly, in girls, the decrease of the AT (-10%) in the same age group exceeds the small but nonsignificant decrease of $\dot{V}O_2$max (-5%). The interaction of changes in $\dot{V}O_2$max and AT (both expressed as mL O_2 • min^{-1} • kg^{-1}) with age results in a significant $(p < .05)$ decrease of AT when expressed as a percent of $\dot{V}O_2$max. The same has been reported by Cooper et al. (1984) in a study of 109 healthy North American boys and girls when the AT/$\dot{V}O_2$max ratio was plotted against body weight $(r = -.28, p < .05)$. This finding suggests an increase in the lactacid anaerobic capacity during growth and confirms earlier observations in kindergarten children where the AT was reached at a higher percent of $\dot{V}O_2$max (mean 67%, Reybrouck et al., 1982) compared to the level in adults (mean 56%, Reybrouck et al., 1983).

Further support for a lower lactacid anaerobic capacity in young children can also be deduced from the lower lactate concentrations measured after maximal exercise in children compared to those in adults (Åstrand, 1952; Davies et al., 1972) and the lower anaerobic capacity measured by the Margaria stair-climbing test (Davies et al., 1972) and the Wingate anaerobic test (Inbar & Bar-Or, 1986). Also, the maximal rate of acidosis after maximal exercise, assessed from the blood pH and base deficit, is not as high in children compared to rates in adolescents and young adults (Bar-Or, 1983; Kinderman, Huber, & Keul, 1975).

This is also confirmed by the shorter O_2 uptake transients in children compared to adults (Cooper, Berry, Lamarra, & Wasserman, 1985; Máček & Vávra, 1980). In studying 10- to 11-year-old boys, Máček and Vávra (1980) observed that the oxygen deficit was smaller than in adults. For an exercise intensity at 90% to 100% of their $\dot{V}O_2$max, boys of 10 to 11 years of age reached 55% of their $\dot{V}O_2$max within 30 s, whereas adults attained only 33% by that time. In addition, the boys needed only 2 min to reach a steady state value, whereas adults needed 3 to 4 min. Other indexes of aerobic function such as the time constant (i.e., the time required to reach 63% of the steady state value for $\dot{V}O_2$) are also correlated with age in girls (Cooper et al., 1985). Older girls (17 years of age) have slower oxygen kinetics than younger girls (9 years of age), but are also less fit. All these data indicate that young children are less capable than adults of performing anaerobic exercise.

Another factor is that, in children, only a very weak correlation $(r = .28$ for boys, $r = .52$ for girls) was found between $\dot{V}O_2$max (mL • min^{-1} • kg^{-1}) and AT (mL • min^{-1} • kg^{-1}). This is at variance with observations in adults where these correlations are much higher (varying from $r = .69$ to $r = .87$; Davis, Frank, Whipp, & Wasserman, 1979; Reybrouck et al., 1983; Reybrouck et al., 1986; Thorland, Sady, & Refsell, 1980; Weltman, Katch, Sadey, & Freedson, 1978). This difference may be explained by the fact that $\dot{V}O_2$max and AT reflect two different physiological mechanisms: $\dot{V}O_2$max is mainly determined by maximal cardiac output and peripheral O_2 extraction (arterio-venous O_2 difference), whereas AT depends to a large extent on the balance between lactate production and lactate removal. One may postulate that, in growing children, the development and maturation of these physiological mechanisms are independent and do not occur at the same rate.

The daily level of physical activity, assessed by a standardized and reproducible questionnaire, was highly correlated with the AT expressed as mL O_2 • min^{-1} • kg^{-1} in boys, but not in girls. When the AT of two activity groups was related to age in boys, the most active boys (51% of the sample) reached the highest value, compared to the less active ones (41% of the sample) at all ages, except in the 12- to 16-year-olds (Figure 5.5). This finding is in agreement with observations of Blimkie, Cunningham, and Nichol (1980), who found similar results for the influence of physical activity on $\dot{V}O_2$max in prepubertal boys. Also, Lange Andersen et al. (1984) found a slight tendency for a higher maximal aerobic power with an increased level of habitual physical activity in adolescent boys. This suggests that during puberty the effect of a high level of daily physical activity on parameters of aerobic function may be masked by other more dominant factors such as hormonal activity, which reaches its maximum during the growth spurt. As healthy girls are physically less active than boys (Ilmarinen & Rutenfranz, 1980; Reybrouck, Weymans, Stijns, & Van der Hauwaert, 1986b), it can be expected that their daily level of physical activity was too low to affect the anaerobic threshold value.

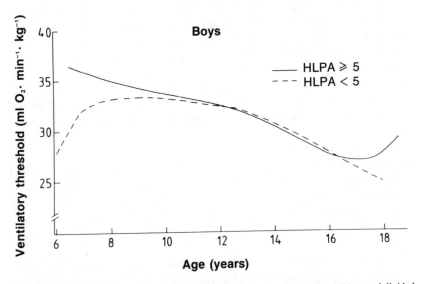

Figure 5.5 Ventilatory anaerobic threshold as a function of age in healthy children, subdivided according to their habitual level of physical activity (HLPA). *Note.* From "Influence of Habitual Levels of Physical Activity on the Cardiorespiratory Endurance Capacity in Children" by M.L. Weymans, T.M. Reybrouck, H.J. Stijns, and J. Knops. In *Children and Exercise XII* (p. 153) by J. Rutenfranz, R. Mocellin, and F. Klimt (Eds.), 1986, Champaign, IL: Human Kinetics. Copyright 1986 by Human Kinetics. Reprinted by permission.

Advantages to and Limitations of Using the Anaerobic Threshold in Pediatric Exercise Testing

Traditionally, maximum aerobic power has been assessed by determination of $\dot{V}O_2$max both in adults (Åstrand & Rodahl, 1977) and in children (Bar-Or, 1983; Cunningham, Paterson, Blimkie, & Donner, 1984). However, a reliable and reproducible measurement of $\dot{V}O_2$max is dependent on the ability to reach a plateau value in $\dot{V}O_2$ during the last loads of an incremental exercise test. In a study on 66 10-year-old boys, Cunningham et al. (1977) demonstrated that only 38% of the boys were able to reach a plateau in $\dot{V}O_2$ at one of two assessments of $\dot{V}O_2$max on a treadmill over a 4- to 5-month period. The maximal endurance time with the Bruce treadmill test has also been used as an index of exercise capacity in children (Cumming, 1978; Cumming, Everatt, & Hastman, 1978), in analogy to its application in adult patients with cardiac disease (Bruce, 1971). However, one of the major drawbacks of this test is its dependence of the child's motivation to perform an all-out effort, which is often low in young children (Godfrey, 1974).

The most precise estimate of AT is obtained by the use of short, incremental exercise tests (1 min per stage; Reybrouck et al., 1983; Wasserman et al., 1986; Whipp, Ward, & Wasserman, 1986), compared to exercise tests with stages of a 4-min duration, which are meant to determine hemodynamic or cardiorespiratory variables under steady state conditions. This is again advantageous for the pediatric age group, because it requires a shorter exercise test.

Because factors other than metabolic acidosis (e.g., anxiety, pain, apprehension) may be responsible for an increased ventilation, particularly in young children, the AT should preferably be determined by not only the disproportionate increase in ventilation relative to $\dot{V}O_2$, but also by measurements of gas exchange that reflect the development of metabolic acidosis (Wasserman, 1983).

Reproducibility of the AT was assessed in 10 pediatric patients varying in age from 9 to 13 years, who were tested twice with a 1-day interval. The test-retest coefficient ($r = .87$) was similar to values reported in the literature for adult subjects, varying from $r = .74$ to $r = .98$ (Caiozzo et al., 1982; Davis et al., 1976; Davis et al., 1979; Hughes et al., 1982; Reybrouck et al., 1983) and even higher than values reported for VO$_2$max in children ($r = .53$; Cunningham et al., 1977).

Under normal conditions, the AT indicates the exercise intensity above which exercise endurance is reduced and tachypnea develops (Jones & Ehrsam, 1982; Reybrouck et al., 1983; Reybrouck et al., 1986; Wasserman et al., 1987). It should be pointed out, however, that occasionally the AT cannot be detected reliably because of an irregular breathing pattern or hyperventilation of a child before the exercise test. For example, we could not determine an AT in 28 out of 283 (10%) healthy children (Reybrouck et al., 1985) and in 4 out of 39 (10%) children who had had operations for tetralogy of Fallot (Reybrouck,

Weymans, Stijns, & Van der Hauwaert, 1986a). In our series of 255 normal children in whom an AT could be identified, the use of the dual criterion (i.e., continuous rise of $\dot{V}_E/\dot{V}O_2$ without a concomitant increase of $\dot{V}_E/\dot{V}CO_2$ could be applied in only 60% of the children. In 31% a disproportionate increase of $\dot{V}_E$ relative to $\dot{V}O_2$ or exercise intensity had to be used. In the remaining 9%, the AT was identified by using the continuous rise of the fractional concentration of O_2 (FEO_2) relative to $\dot{V}O_2$.

Similar to observations made in adults (Davis et al., 1979), the AT measurement is a sensitive index of training specialty in children. In a study on 54 eleven-year-old boys, Vanden Eynde and Van Coppenolle (1988) found that boys who were specifically trained for sprinting had a significantly lower value for AT, expressed as a percentage of $\dot{V}O_2$max, compared to endurance runners and controls (Figure 5.6). Although this is a cross-sectional comparison, it is possible that the AT in children may be sensitive to specific training effects.

CLINICAL APPLICABILITY OF THE ANAEROBIC THRESHOLD IN PEDIATRIC EXERCISE TESTING

In clinical exercise testing of 50 children with congenital heart disease and a left-to-right shunt (ventricular septal defect, $n = 43$: atrial septal defect, $n = 7$), we found the AT measurement more sensitive in detecting subnormal exercise performance than other, still widely used, indexes of exercise performance capacity, such as the oxygen uptake reached at a heart rate of

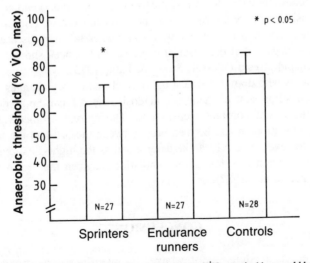

Figure 5.6 Anaerobic threshold (expressed as a percentage of $\dot{V}O_2$max in 11-year-old boys specifically trained for sprint and endurance running, compared to controls. *Note*. Data courtesy of Dr. B. Vanden Eynde.

170 beats • min^{-1} ($\dot{V}O_2$170; Reybrouck et al., 1986b). In this series, twice as many patients showed a subnormal value (below the 95% confidence limit) for AT (56%) than for the $\dot{V}O_2$170 test (28%; Figure 5.7). The difference was statistically significant ($p < .05$). When expressed as a percentage of the age- and sex-predicted normal values, the mean AT (89.1 $\pm$ 14.4%) was significantly ($p < .001$) lower than the mean $\dot{V}O_2$170 (103 $\pm$ 17.2%). A subnormal cardiorespiratory endurance capacity in a large portion of these patients was associated with a reduced level of daily physical activity, as generally observed in children with congenital heart disease (Bar-Or, 1983; Strong & Alpert, 1982). Furthermore, in children operated on for tetralogy of Fallot, a lower than normal heart rate response to exercise was found in about half of the patients, and the $\dot{V}O_2$170 was normal (Reybrouck et al., 1986a). Theoretically, these findings could be interpreted as indicting a normal or high physical performance capacity. In contrast, however, the mean AT was significantly different and averaged 89.3 $\pm$ 15.7% of age-predicted normal value. These examples show that the use of AT measurement in pediatric patients is more sensitive in discriminating subnormal exercise capacity from normal standards. In addition, its measurement is independent of heart rate response. We therefore recommend evaluating cardiorespiratory exercise performance capacity by not only measuring heart rate response, but also analyzing gas exchange during exercise.

In adult patients with marked airway obstruction, it has been shown that the AT usually cannot be determined by gas exchange methods, because of the onset of dyspnea at very low exercise levels (Nery et al., 1982; Wasserman et al., 1987). In children with low breathing reserve, such as in severe cystic fibrosis or asthma, AT measurement may be difficult or impossible to determine, because they develop a progressive degree of hyperventilation at very low intensities of exercise or even at the onset of exercise (Godfrey, 1974). Difficulties may also arise in children with congenital heart disease when AT is already surpassed at the onset of exercise, as has been shown in children with tricuspid atresia (Wessel, Stout, & Paul, 1985).

In patients who do not manifest the normal ventilatory changes associated with the development of metabolic acidosis, the AT can be ascertained by performing several constant intensity tests. During such protocols, the difference in ventilation should be measured between the 3rd and the 6th min of an exercise level. The AT can be determined as the highest exercise level at which no difference is found for ventilation between the 3rd and 6th min (Wasserman et al., 1987).

CONCLUSION

In children, as in adults, a critical exercise intensity can be shown at which a concomitant disproportionate increase in pulmonary ventilation and plasma lactate occurs relative to oxygen uptake. This has been defined as the *anaerobic*

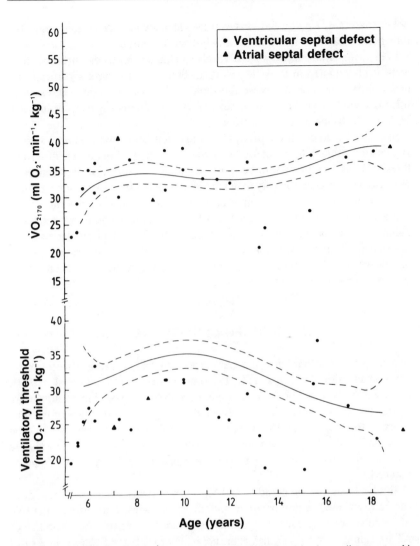

Figure 5.7   Individual values for V̇O₂ at a heart rate of 170 bpm and for the ventilatory anaerobic threshold plotted against the 95% confidence limits of the normal values in boys. *Note.* From "Ventilatory Anaerobic Threshold for Evaluating Exercise Performance in Children With Congenital Left-to-Right Intracardiac Shunt" by T. Reybrouck, M. Weymans, H. Stijns, and L.G. Van der Hauwaert, 1986, *Pediatric Cardiology,* 7, p. 21. Copyright 1986 by Pediatric Cardiology. Reprinted by permission.

threshold and represents the exercise intensity above which exercise is difficult to maintain because of the accumulation of lactate.

Although a cause-and-effect relationship between onset of plasma lactate accumulation and disproportionate increase in ventilation, relative to V̇O₂, is not yet definitely established, this exercise intensity has been called anaerobic threshold because it is the most widely used definition.

In growing children, boys have a higher value for anaerobic threshold than girls at all ages (from 6 to 18 years). In both sex groups, a significant decrease was found for anaerobic threshold with advancing age, expressed as mL O_2 • min^{-1} • kg^{-1} or as a percent of $\dot{V}O_2$max. This suggests an increase with age in lactacid anaerobic capacity.

In clinical studies on children with congenital heart disease and a left-to-right shunt, or in children after total repair of tetralogy of Fallot, the anaerobic threshold has been shown to be more sensitive in discriminating subnormal exercise performance capacity than other still widely used criteria such as heart rate response (e.g., power output at a heart rate of 170 beats • min^{-1}).

It is concluded that the AT can be easily determined in children when using parameters of gas exchange during exercise. This is particularly useful in the assessment of cardiorespiratory endurance capacity in the pediatric age group, because it is independent of the child's motivation to perform exercise, as required for maximal exercise testing.

CHALLENGES FOR FUTURE RESEARCH

In adult patients with cardiopulmonary disease that significantly affects cardiovascular function (Sietsema et al., 1986) or gas exchange (Nery et al., 1982), the rise of $\dot{V}O_2$ at the start of exercise has been shown to be slowed at exercise intensities below the AT. This is reflected in a significant increase of the time constant for $\dot{V}O_2$ (i.e., 63% of the time required to attain a steady state). The same studies should be done in pediatric patients with cardiopulmonary disease to understand why exercise performance capacity, assessed by AT, may be reduced.

Similar to studies on heredity and $\dot{V}O_2$max in twins, measurements of AT can be performed in homozygotic and dizygotic twins to investigate the role of heredity on their cardiorespiratory endurance capacity. An advantage of AT measurement over $\dot{V}O_2$max is the possibility to define it from a submaximal exercise test, which makes it independent of the child's motivation to perform maximal exercise testing.

Although it is more difficult to take blood samples in children, more data are needed on blood lactate in children to study the relationship between changes in blood lactate and alterations in gas exchange. This should be studied in a variety of experimental conditions.

Finally, little is known about the longitudinal influence of growth and training on AT in children and whether AT changes in the same way after training, as has been reported for adults (Davis et al., 1979). Further experiments on the influence of training are desirable.

ACKNOWLEDGMENTS

Work related to this chapter was performed in collaboration with A. Amery, R. Fagard, J. Ghesquiere, J. Faulkner, L. Van der Hauwaert, and M. Weymans. We gratefully acknowledge the help of Mrs. Daniëlle Priem and Miss Hilde Vuerinckx in preparing and typing this manuscript.

REFERENCES

Åstrand, P.O. (1952). *Experimental studies of physical working capacity in relation to sex and age.* Copenhagen: Ejnar Munksgaard.

Åstrand, P.O., & Rodahl, K. (1977). *Textbook of work physiology* (2nd Ed.). New York: McGraw Hill.

Bar-Or. (1983). *Pediatric sports medicine for the practitioner.* New York: Springer-Verlag.

Blimkie, C.J.R., Cunningham, D.J., & Nichol , M.M. (1980). Gas transport capacity and echocardiographically determined cardiac size in children. *Journal of Applied Physiology,* **49**, 994-999.

Brooks, G.A. (1985). Anaerobic threshold: Review of the concept and directions for future research. *Medicine and Science in Sports and Exercise,* **17**, 22-31.

Bruce, R.A. (1971). Exercise testing of patients with coronary heart disease. Principles and normal standards for evaluation. *Annals of Clinical Research,* **3**, 323-332.

Caiozzo, V.J., Davis, J.A., Ellis, J.F., Azus, J.L., Vandagriff, R., Prietto, C.A., & McMaster, W.C. (1982). A comparison of gas exchange indices used to detect the anaerobic threshold. *Journal of Applied Physiology,* **53**, 1184-1189.

Cooper, D.M., Berry, C., Lamarra, N., & Wasserman, K. (1985). Kinetics of oxygen uptake and heart rate at onset of exercise in children. *Journal of Applied Physiology,* **59**, 211-217.

Cooper, D.M., Weiler-Ravell, D., Whipp, B.J., & Wasserman, K. (1984). Aerobic parameters of exercise as a function of body size during growth in children. *Journal of Applied Physiology,* **56**, 628-634.

Cumming, G.R. (1978). Maximal exercise capacity of children with heart defects. *American Journal of Cardiology,* **42**, 613-619.

Cumming, G.R., Everatt, D., & Hastman, L. (1978). Bruce treadmill test in children: Normal values in a clinic population. *American Journal of Cardiology,* **41**, 69-75.

Cunningham, D.A., Paterson, D.H., Blimkie, C.J.R., & Donner, A.P. (1984). Development of cardiorespiratory function in circumpubertal boys: A longitudinal study. *Journal of Applied Physiology,* **56**, 302-307.

Cunningham, D.A., Van Waterschoot, B., Paterson, D.H., Lefcoe, M., & Sangal, S.P. (1977). Reliability and reproducibility of maximal oxygen uptake measurements in children. *Medicine and Science in Sports,* **9**, 104-108.

Davies, C.T.M., Barnes, C., & Godfrey, S. (1972). Body composition and maximal exercise performance in children. *Human Biology,* **44**, 195-214.

Davis, J.A. (1985). Anaerobic threshold: Review of the concept and directions for future research. *Medicine and Science in Sports and Exercise,* **17**, 6-18.

Davis, J.A., Frank, M.H., Whipp, B.J., & Wasserman, K. (1979). Anaerobic threshold alterations caused by endurance training in middle-aged men. *Journal of Applied Physiology,* **46**, 1039-1046.

Davis, J.A., Vodak, P., Wilmore, J.H., Vodak, J., & Kurtz, P. (1976). Anaerobic threshold and maximal aerobic power for three modes of exercise. *Journal of Applied Physiology,* **41**, 544-550.

Eriksson, B.O. (1972). Physical training, oxygen supply and muscle metabolism in 11-13 year old boys. *Acta Physiologica Scandinavica,* **86**(Suppl. 384), 1-48.

Eriksson, B.O., & Koch, G. (1973). Effects of physical training on haemodynamic response during submaximal and maximal exercise in 11-13 year old boys. *Acta Physiologica Scandinavica,* **87**, 27-39.

Gadhoke, S., & Jones, N.L. (1973). The response to exercise in boys aged 9-15 years. *Clinical Science,* **37**, 789-801.

Gaisl, G., & Buchberger, J. (1982). Veränderungen des aerob-anaeroben Übergangs bei 13- bis 14 jährigen Sportschülern nach 3 Jahren Training [Changes in aerobic-anaerobic transition, in 13-14 year old schoolchildren, after 3 years of training]. *Leistungssport,* **12**, 62-66.

Gaisl, G., & Wiesspeiner, G. (1986). Training prescriptions for 9- to 17-year-old figure skaters based on lactate assessment in the laboratory and on the ice. In J. Rutenfranz, R. Mocellin, & F. Klimt (Eds.), *Children and exercise* (Vol. 12, pp. 59-60). Champaign, IL: Human Kinetics.

Gladden, B.L. (1984). Current "anaerobic threshold" controversies. *The Physiologist,* **27**, 312-317.

Godfrey, S. (1974). *Exercise testing in children.* London: Saunders.

Gollnick, P.D., Armstrong, R.B., Saubert I.V.C., Piehl, K., & Saltin, B. (1972). Enzyme activity and fiber composition in skeletal muscle of untrained and trained men. *Journal of Applied Physiology,* **33**, 312-319.

Hughes, E., Turner, S.C., & Brooks, G.A. (1982). Effects of glycogen depletion and pedalling speed on "anaerobic threshold." *Journal of Applied Physiology,* **52,** 1598-1607.

Ilmarinen, J., & Rutenfranz, J. (1980). Longitudinal studies of the changes in habitual physical activity of schoolchildren and working adolescents. In K. Berg & B. O. Eriksson (Eds.), *Children and exercise* (Vol. 9, pp. 149-159). Baltimore: University Park Press.

Inbar, O., & Bar-Or, O. (1986). Anaerobic characteristics in male children and adolescents. *Medicine and Science in Sports and Exercise,* **18,** 264-269.

Jones, N.L., & Ehrsam, R.E. (1982). The anaerobic threshold. *Exercise and Sport Sciences Reviews,* **10,** 49-83.

Kinderman, W., Huber, G., & Keul, J. (1975). Anaerobic Kapazität bei Kindern und Jugenlichen in Beziehung zum Erwacksenen [Anaerobic capacity in children and adolescents compared to adults]. *Sportarzt und Sportmedizin,* **6,** 112-115.

Kinderman, W., Simon, G., & Keul, J. (1979). The significance of the aerobic-anaerobic transition for the determination of work load intensities during endurance training. *European Journal of Applied Physiology,* **42,** 25-34.

Kremser, C.B., & Rajfer, S.I. (1986). The normal cardiovascular response to exercise. In A.R. Leff (Ed.), *Cardiopulmonary exercise testing* (pp. 107-122). Orlando: Grune & Stratton.

Lange Andersen, K.L., Ilmarinen, J., Rutenfranz, J., Ottmann, W., Berndt, J., Kylian, H., & Ruppel, M. (1984). Leisure time sports activities and maximal aerobic power during late adolescence. *European Journal of Applied Physiology,* **52,** 431-436.

Máček, M., & Vávra, J. (1969). Aerobic and anaerobic metabolism during exercise in childhood. *Mallati Cardiovasculari,* **10,** 409-420.

Máček, M., & Vávra, J. (1971). Cardiopulmonary and metabolic changes during exercise in children 6-14 years old. *Journal of Applied Physiology,* **30,** 202-204.

Máček, M., & Vávra, J. (1980). the adjustment of oxygen uptake at the onset of exercise: A comparison between prepubertal boys and young adults. *International Journal of Sports Medicine,* **1,** 75-77.

Máček, M., & Vávra, J. (1985). Anaerobic threshold in children. In R.A. Binkhorst, H.C.G. Kemper, & W.H.M. Saris (Eds.), *Children and exercise* (Vol. 11, pp. 110-113). Champaign, IL: Human Kinetics.

Mader, A., Liesen, H., Heck, H., Philippi, H., Rost, R., Schürch, P., & Hollmann, W. (1976). Zur beurteilung der sportartspezifischen Ausdauerleistungsfähigkeit in Labor [Assessment of endurance performance capacity related to sportdisciplines]. *Sportarzt und Sportmedizin,* **27,** 109-112.

Margaria, R. (1979). *Biomechanics and energetics of muscular exercise.* Oxford: Clarendon.

McLellan, T.M. (1985). Ventilatory and plasma lactate response with different exercise protocols: A comparison of methods. *International Journal of Sports Medicine,* **6**, 30-35.

Nery, L.E., Wasserman, K., Andrews, J.A., Huntsman, D.J., Hansen, J.E., & Whipp, B.J. (1982). Ventilatory and gas exchange kinetics during exercise in chronic airway obstruction. *Journal of Applied Physiology,* **53**, 1594-1597.

Reybrouck, T., Ghesquiere, J., Cattaert, A., Fagard, R., & Amery, A. (1983). Ventilatory thresholds during short- and long-term exercise. *Journal of Applied Physiology,* **55**, 1694-1700.

Reybrouck, T., Ghesquiere, J., Weymans, M., & Amery, A. (1986). Ventilatory threshold measurement to evaluate maximal endurance performance. *International Journal of Sports Medicine,* **7**, 26-29.

Reybrouck, T., Weymans, M., Ghesquiere, J., Van Gerven, D., & Stijns, H. (1982). Ventilatory threshold during treadmill exercise in kindergarten children. *European Journal of Applied Physiology,* **50**, 79-86.

Reybrouck, T., Weymans, M., Stijns, H., Knops, J., & Van der Hauwaert, L. (1985). Ventilatory anaerobic threshold in healthy children: Age and sex differences. *European Journal of Applied Physiology,* **54**, 278-284.

Reybrouck, T., Weymans, M., Stijns, H., Van der Hauwaert, L.G. (1986a). Exercise testing after correction of tetralogy of Fallot: The fallacy of a reduced heart rate response. *American Heart Journal,* **112**, 998-1003.

Reybrouck, T., Weymans, M., Stijns, H., & Van der Hauwaert, L.G. (1986b). Ventilatory anaerobic threshold for evaluating exercise performance in children with congenital left-to-right intracardiac shunt. *Pediatric Cardiology,* **7**, 19-24.

Sietsema, K.E., Cooper, D.M., Perloff, J.K., Rosove, M.H., Child, J.S., Canobbio, M.M., Whipp, B.J., & Wasserman, K. (1986). Dynamics of oxygen uptake during exercise in adults with cyanotic congenital heart disease. *Circulation,* **73**, 1137-1144.

Stremel, R.W. (1984). Historical development of the anaerobic threshold concept. *Physiologist,* **27**, 295-297.

Strong, W.B., & Alpert, B.S. (1982). The child with heart disease: Current problems in pediatrics. *Year Book Medical,* 1-34.

Tavazzi, I., & di Prampero, P.E. (Eds.). (1986). *The anaerobic threshold: Physiological and clinical significance.* Basel, Switzerland: Karger.

Thorland, W.S., Sady, S., & Refsell, M. (1980). Anaerobic threshold and maximum oxygen consumption rates as predictors of cross country running performance. *Medicine and Science in Sports and Exercise,* **12**, 87.

Vanden Eynde, B., & Van Coppenolle, A. (1988). *Effects of specific training in children on maximal aerobic power and anaerobic threshold.* Unpublished manuscript, University of Leuven, Leuven, Belgium.

Wasserman, K. (1983). Misconceptions and missed perceptions of the anaerobic threshold [Letter to the editor]. *Journal of Applied Physiology, 53,* 853-854.

Wasserman, K. (1984). The anaerobic threshold measurement to evaluate exercise performance. *American Review of Respiratory Disease, 129,* 535-540.

Wasserman, K., Hansen, J., Sue, D.Y., & Whipp, B.J. (1987). *Principles of exercise testing and interpretation.* Philadelphia: Lea & Febiger.

Wasserman, K., & Whipp, B.J. (1975). Exercise physiology in health and disease. *American Review of Respiratory Disease, 112,* 219-249.

Wasserman, K., Whipp, B.J., Koyal, N.S., & Beaver, W.L. (1973). Anaerobic threshold and respiratory gas exchange during exercise. *Journal of Applied Physiology, 35,* 236-243.

Weltman, A., Katch, V., Sadey, S., & Freedson, P. (1978). Onset of anaerobic metabolism (anaerobic threshold) as a criterion measure of submaximum fitness. *Research Quarterly, 48,* 218-227.

Wessel, H.U., Stout, R.L., & Paul, M.H. (1985). Exercise in postoperative tricuspid atresia. In R.A. Binkhorst, H.C.G. Kemper, & W.H.M. Saris (Eds.), *Children and exercise* (Vol. 11, pp. 93-99). Champaign, IL: Human Kinetics.

Weymans, M.L., Reybrouck, T.M., Stijns, H.J., & Knops, J. (1986). Influence of habitual levels of physical activity on the cardiorespiratory endurance capacity in children. In J. Rutenfranz, R. Mocellin, & F. Klimt (Eds.), *Children and exercise* (Vol. 12, pp. 149-156). Champaign, IL: Human Kinetics.

Whipp, B.J., Davis, J.A., Torres, F., & Wasserman, K. (1981). A test to determine parameters of aerobic function. *Journal of Applied Physiology, 50,* 217-221.

Whipp, B.J., Ward, S.A., & Wasserman, K. (1986). Respiratory markers of the anaerobic threshold. In L. Tavazzi & P.E. di Prampero (Eds.), *The anaerobic threshold: Physiological and clinical significance* (pp. 47-64). Basel, Switzerland: Karger.

6

Rating of Perceived Exertion in Children

Oded Bar-Or
McMaster University, Hamilton, Ontario, Canada
Dianne S. Ward
University of South Carolina

In 1962 Borg suggested, for the first time, the relevance of psychophysical principles to the *rating of perceived exertion* (RPE). Since then, much knowledge has been generated regarding the manner in which people rate the intensity of their physical effort and the possible mechanisms and pathways by which such effort is perceived. Borg's (1970) 6-to-20 category scale and, more recently (Borg, 1982), a zero-to-maximum ratio-category scale have been used by psychophysicists, physiologists, psychologists, and clinicians in research, assessment of fitness, and rehabilitation. The vast majority of these observations has been related to adults.

Relatively little information is available on the way children and adolescents rate the intensity of their effort. The purpose of this chapter is to review this information. Specifically, we focus on possible age- and maturation-related differences in rating of exercise intensity by healthy populations. We describe changes in RPE of children who undergo conditioning or heat acclimation, the RPE of the child with a disease, and the possible use of RPE in prescription of exercise for healthy or disabled children.

RPE AT DIFFERENT AGES

In constructing his 6-to-20 category scale, Borg chose rating numbers that would increase linearly with the intensity of exercise. The physiologic index chosen by Borg to reflect exercise intensity was heart rate (HR), which, at a wide range of submaximal efforts, is linear with exercise intensity (e.g., mechanical power on the cycle ergometer). Specifically, the rating numbers were selected to correspond, in adults, to approximately 1/10 of the HR at any given submaximal effort. Thus, when a person exerts at an intensity that he or she rates as 15 (i.e., hard), his or her HR will be about 150 beat • min^{-1}. This 1:10 ratio between RPE and HR seemed, by and large, to hold for young adults and middle-aged people at various levels of fitness and body adiposity, as well as in several climatic conditions and modes of exercise (e.g., Bar-Or, Skinner, Buskirk, & Borg, 1972; Carton & Rhodes, 1985; Skinner, Borg, & Buskirk, 1969; Skinner, Hustler, Bergsteinová, & Buskirk, 1973a, 1973b), suggesting a consistent association between RPE and physiologic strain.

Does this ratio hold true for children? In a cross-sectional study of 1,316 seven- to sixty-eight-year-old Israeli males, Bar-Or (1977) discovered that, at any given HR level, children rated their exercise intensity lower than adolescents, who, in turn, rated it lower than adults. As shown in Figure 6.1, the RPE/HR ratio in 10-year-old boys was only 0.7:10 and at age 13 it was 0.8:10. One exception to that pattern was a group of 7- to 9-year-old gymnasts whose ratio was close to 1:10.

It might be argued that, because maximal HR is higher in children than in adults, a certain submaximal HR denotes a lower physiologic strain in the child. A better index of physiologic strain, therefore, would be the percentage of maximal HR (%HRmax). One can assume that a certain %HRmax denotes a similar physiologic strain in a child, an adolescent, and a young adult. Figure 6.2 summarizes data from five studies, relating the ratio RPE/%HRmax to age. There are 16 data points on the graph, each representing a mean value for a certain age group at exercise intensities of 70%-80% peak aerobic power. It is apparent that, at any given physiologic strain, children rate their exercise intensity lower than adolescents or young adults.

The reason for such low rating in children is hard to interpret, mostly because one does not yet understand the mechanisms for RPE (Cafarelli, 1982; Carton & Rhodes, 1985; Pandolf, 1982; Robertson, 1982). The data in Figure 6.2 were obtained using the scale in four languages (English, Finnish, Arabic, and Hebrew). It is, therefore, unlikely that these age-related differences are due to semantic interpretation of the RPE scale. RPE in children (Rutenfranz,

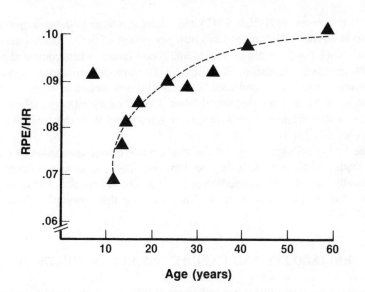

Figure 6.1   Age-group means for RPE/HR in 7- to 68-year-old men *(N* = 1,316) at a 100-W work load during a progressive test on the cycle ergometer (line drawn by eyeball approximation). *Note*. From "Age-Related Changes in Exercise Perception" (p. 261) by O. Bar-Or. Reprinted with permission from G. Borg (Ed.), *Physical Work and Effort*, copyright 1977, Pergamon Books Ltd.

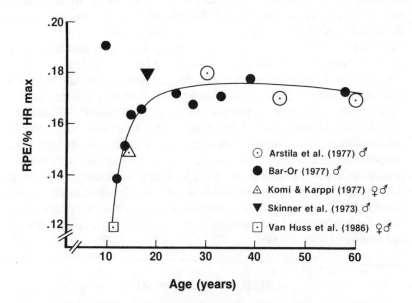

Figure 6.2   Age-group means for RPE/%HRmax at different ages using data from Figure 6.1 and four other studies (line drawn by eyeball approximation).

Klimt, Ilmarinen, & Kylian, 1977) and adults is related to the concentration of blood lactate. Children, at any given percentage of their maximal aerobic power, have lower levels of muscle and blood lactate when compared with adults (Eriksson, Karlsson, & Saltin, 1971). Although no cause-and-effect relationship has been established between RPE and lactate levels (Carton & Rhodes, 1985), it is possible that children's lower rating reflects a lower reliance on anaerobic energy pathways at any given intensity of submaximal exercise (Bar-Or, 1983).

The biological significance of children's relative underestimation of effort is a matter of conjecture. It may be, however, one reason why children are habitually more active than adolescents and adults. It may also reflect the old adage that parents tire more easily from watching their child play than does the child itself.

RELIABILITY AND VALIDITY OF RPE IN CHILDREN

In adults, test-retest reliability coefficients of RPE at a given exercise intensity have ranged from .70 to .90 (e.g., Carton & Rhodes, 1985; Skinner et al., 1973b; Stamford, 1976). Similar r values have been found among children (Kahle, Ulmer, & Rummel, 1977; Ward & Bar-Or, 1987; Ward, Blimkie, & Bar-Or, 1986), particularly at intensities higher than 50% of maximal aerobic power (Komi & Karppi, 1977; Ward & Bar-Or, 1987). Good reproducibility, as determined by similarity of RPE values in repeated testing, has been shown for children and adolescents (Komi & Karppi, 1977; Ward & Bar-Or, in press. Kahle et al. (1977), who studied 7- to 11-year-old females, stated that the test-retest reproducibility in the youngest age group was higher than in the older children. However, no data were provided for each age group.

No cause-and-effect relationship can be implied between RPE and HR. However, the strength of association between the two variables has been taken to represent the validity or accuracy of rating (e.g., Miyashita, Onodera, & Tabata, 1986; Skinner et al., 1973b; Ulmer, Janz, & Lollgen, 1977). Numerous studies have been conducted on adults that have analyzed the RPE to HR relationship. This has also been the approach in most studies with children. In general, authors agree that the validity of RPE in children, based on the RPE to HR (or %HRmax) correlation, is not lower than that found in adults (Bar-Or, 1977; Miyashita et al., 1986; Ward et al., 1986). For more discussion of this relationship, see sections in this chapter on critical age, obesity, and neuromuscular disease.

CRITICAL AGE FOR RPE

What is the youngest age below which a child cannot rate her or his exercise intensity with high enough validity? This question was addressed recently by

Miyashita et al. (1986), who tested 120 seven- to eighteen-year-old Japanese boys. Although the RPE versus %HRmax correlation coefficients were consistently above .90 in the boys 10 years old and older, they were only .55-.74 in the 7- to 9-year-olds. The authors concluded that the critical age for understanding the (Japanese) RPE scale was 9 years. A similar trend was obtained in the Israeli study by Bar-Or (1977), where the RPE versus HR correlation coefficients in 7- to 9-year-old gymnasts were lower than in the older children and adolescents. RPE has been documented routinely in the Children's Exercise and Nutrition Centre in Hamilton, Canada. It is seldom that a child who is younger than 8 years can give a reasonable rating (i.e., one that increases linearly with exercise intensity). In their study of 7- to 11-year-old German females, Kahle et al. (1977) stated that "rating of perceived exertion is based on a learning process while maturing" (p. R28). Yet, they have not provided any data of the validity of RPE in these subjects.

A question arises as to whether young children can process numbers and assign them to physical events of a known magnitude. As reported by Teghstoonian (cited in Borg, 1977), 8- and 9-year-old children were able to assign numbers to sound pressure levels in a manner and variability similar to those found in older children and adults.

More studies are indicated to systematically address the issue of critical age for valid RPE in girls and boys. Most likely it is the mental age, rather than the chronological age, that determines one's ability to rate exercise intensity. Another issue that merits further research and development is the possibility that descriptors other than numbers (e.g., graphic figures and symbols) can be used with young children to rate their perceived exertion.

RPE IN THE CHILD WITH DISEASE

Obesity

Many professionals in the field of physical education and exercise intuitively feel that overweight and obese children and adolescents cannot or do not evaluate levels of physical exertion accurately. Perhaps this assumption is based on observations of the exercise behavior of these young people. In physical education classes, for example, obese children often are found on the periphery of group activity, and some withdraw from participation altogether. This behavior, as well as verbal complaints, leads one to hypothesize that the obese child might inappropriately consider physical activity as too difficult.

Little work has been done on the use of RPE with obese adults and even less with obese children. Bar-Or et al. (1972) and Skinner et al. (1973a) found that the degree of adiposity did not interfere with the ability of adults to rate their physical effort accurately. The consistency of this finding with children and adolescents was recently studied. Ward et al. (1986) compared the rating by 43 obese outpatient adolescents to that of a reference group of 50 healthy high school students. RPE, based on the Borg category scale, was monitored during progressive maximal cycling. When calculated at any given level of mechanical power, RPE in the obese children was some 1.5-2.5 units higher than in the reference group. However, when this comparison was adjusted to account for fitness levels (relating RPE to % peak power), differences between the groups decreased to about one RPE unit. Although this latter difference was statistically significant, the biological significance, if any, of one RPE unit is unclear.

Table 6.1 is a summary of the correlation coefficients between RPE and objective indexes of effort in the obese children from the study described, as well as for those with other diseases and healthy ones. As shown for adults, the association of RPE with % peak power was stronger than with absolute power or HR. There were no differences in these indexes of validity between the obese and the healthy children.

Table 6.1   Correlation Coefficients Between RPE and Objective Indexes of Effort Intensity in Girls (F) and Boys (M) With a Disease and in a Healthy Comparison Group

Group	Number of observations	Limbs	HR	Power	% peak power
Obesity					
F	21	Lower	0.72	0.71	0.84
M	12	Lower	0.80	0.74	0.84
Muscular dystrophy/atrophy					
M	13	Upper	0.69	0.80	0.92
M	40	Lower	0.72	0.53	0.79
F	22	Lower	0.69	0.69	0.72
Spina bifida					
F	14	Upper	0.82	0.48	0.80
M	20	Upper	0.58	0.73	0.74
Cerebral palsy					
F	25	Lower	0.78	0.66	0.86
M	21	Lower	0.77	0.12	0.68
Healthy					
F	89	Upper	0.78	0.82	0.91
M	100	Upper	0.81	0.87	0.86
F	141	Lower	0.69	0.74	0.79
M	122	Lower	0.82	0.77	0.86

Note. Data from Bar-Or and Reed, 1986; Ward, Blimkie, and Bar-Or, 1986.

Eleven of the obese adolescents in the Ward et al. (1986) study were retested within a 4-month period. Although mean rating in Test 1 was somewhat higher than in Test 2 (12.9 vs. 12.0, $p > .05$), the test-retest correlation was .92.

In another study (Ward & Bar-Or, 1987), 20 obese children were asked to rate four, 2-min submaximal work loads using the Borg 6-to-20 category scale. Two days later, the protocol was repeated. Subjects were not aware of the purpose of the study. Test-retest correlation coefficients ranged from .59 at the lowest intensity (20% peak power) to .89 at the highest load (80% peak power). This pattern was apparent whether intensities were presented in a progressive (stepwise) manner or in a random sequence.

From these observations it can be concluded that obese children can rate their perceived exercise intensity *accurately* and *consistently*. Even though they assign a high rating to a given effort, their rating per percentage of maximal aerobic power is similar to that of the general child population. When an obese child complains that an exercise task is too strenuous, perhaps the exercise therapist should pay closer attention to this complaint. It may reflect a true higher physiologic strain, rather than an exaggerated rating.

Anorexia Nervosa

Anorexia nervosa (AN) is an eating disorder that is often accompanied by an excessive and compulsive activity pattern. It has been suggested that patients with AN display denial of exertion and of postexertional fatigue (Dally, 1969), which may cause them to underestimate the intensity of exertion experienced. This might be reflected by underestimation of RPE. Davies, Fohlin, and Thorén (1980) compared the rating of nine 12- to 18-year-old AN patients and eight controls during a 60-min steady state cycling test at 61%-66% maximal aerobic power. RPE at 10 min was 13.0 in the patients and 12.6 in the controls. At 60 min, the respective values were 15.1 and 13.7. These intergroup differences were nonsignificant. The results of this study do not confirm the notion that teenagers with AN have an impaired ability to rate their perceived exertion.

Neuromuscular Disease

Very little information is available on the rating of perceived exertion in adult patients who suffer from a neuromuscular or skeletal disease (Birk et al., 1983; Bjuro, Fugl-Meyer, Grimby, Hook, & Lundgren, 1975; Nordemar, Edstrom, & Ekblom, 1976). As a general rule, these patients have a low level of fitness and, as shown by Bjuro et al. (1975) for hemiplegics and those with multiple sclerosis, their RPE at any given exercise intensity is high. Sargeant and Davies (1977) compared young adults who sustained muscle atrophy due to immobilization following leg fracture to healthy controls. Although the patients rated higher at any given exercise intensity, the rating at a certain percentage of maximal aerobic power was identical. The same authors have shown in previous work with healthy adults that, irrespective of the mass of the muscle that performs an activity, RPE is the same when exercise intensity is described as percentage of maximal aerobic power (determined during exercise with the respective muscle group).

We are familiar with only one study in which RPE was assessed in children and adolescents with a neuromuscular disease (Bar-Or & Reed, 1986). These were 10- to 20-year-old girls and boys *(N* = 24) with spastic cerebral palsy, spina bifida, myopathy, muscular dystrophy, and muscular atrophy. Their response to cycling or arm cranking was compared to that of 101 healthy controls. Figures 6.3 and 6.4 summarize the results for the girls who performed the leg exercise. Although most of the patients had a higher than normal RPE at any given *absolute* power level, their ratings were virtually identical to those of the controls when plotted against % peak power. Similar findings were evident for arm exercise and for females and males, alike. Correlation coefficients between RPE and some objective indexes of exercise intensity are shown in Table 6.1. As found for healthy and for obese children, *r* values were consistently higher in the children with neuromuscular disease when related to % peak power than to absolute power or HR. Correlations between RPE and % peak power ranged from .68 to .92 and were similar across diagnostic groups.

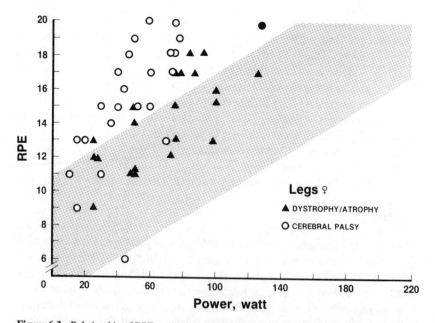

Figure 6.3 Relationship of RPE to absolute mechanical power during cycling exercise in female children and adolescents with neuromuscular disease (gray area represents the 95% confidence range for 50 healthy high school females). *Note.* From "Rating of Perceived Exertion of Adolescents With Neuromuscular Disease" by O. Bar-Or and S.L. Reed, 1986, in G. Borg and D. Ottoson (Eds.), *The Perception of Exertion in Physical Work* (p. 140), Basingstoke, England: Macmillan. Copyright 1986 by Macmillan. Reprinted by permission of Macmillan, London and Basingstoke.

Although the mechanisms for perception of exercise intensity are not clear, it seems that, in part, they involve proprioceptive and other cues from the

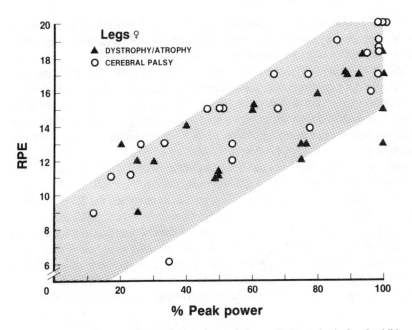

Figure 6.4 Relationship of RPE to % peak power during cycling exercise in female children and adolescents with neuromuscular disease (subjects and symbols as in Figure 6.3). *Note*. From "Rating of Perceived Exertion of Adolescents With Neuromuscular Disease" by O. Bar-Or and S.L. Reed, 1986, in G. Borg and D. Ottoson (Eds.), *The Perception of Exertion in Physical Work* (p. 141), Basingstoke, England: Macmillan. Copyright 1986 by Macmillan. Reprinted by permission of Macmillan, London and Basingstoke.

exercising muscles, tendons, and joints. The intensity of such cues apparently depends on the strain experienced by the muscles and the joints (Pandolf, 1982). The described regularity in rating, irrespective of the type of neuromuscular disease, is somewhat surprising. It is implausible that exercise-related peripheral signals are equally intact in healthy limbs and in those with markedly atrophic, dystrophic, or spastic muscles. The near uniform RPE in all these groups, therefore, lends support to the notion that central, and not only peripheral, cues trigger one's exercise perception. The findings cited are in line with those described by Cafarelli (1982), who used a matching muscle model, and they support the notion that exercise intensity is perceived through not only feedback from the periphery, but also a feedforward loop.

EFFECTS OF TRAINING AND ACCLIMATION TO HEAT

Many studies with adults have shown that training induces a reduction in RPE for a given exercise intensity. Several (Docktor & Sharkey, 1971; Ekblom & Goldbarg, 1971; Kilbom, 1971; Miyashita et al., 1986), but not all (Pandolf,

Burse, & Goldman, 1975), studies demonstrated that, although aerobic training is accompanied by a reduction in both RPE and HR, the RPE on HR regression line does not change. In a study performed at the Wingate Institute in Israel (Bar-Or & Inbar, 1977), eight 8- to 10-year-old boys were trained in a thermo-neutral indoor environment (six sessions of cycling for 60 min at 40%-50% maximal oxygen uptake during a 2-week period). Nine other boys and nine 20- to 23-year-old men underwent a heat acclimation program, in which they trained in a similar protocol, but at 43 °C, 55% relative humidity. Control groups of children ($N = 7$) and young adults ($N = 7$) were tested before and after the 2-week period but did not train. As expected, both the training and the acclimation groups had a gradual reduction in their HR and RPE. The controls had no change in either. Figure 6.5 summarizes the RPE/HR ratio as determined at the end of each training session. A marked difference is seen between the perceptual response to training in the children and in a comparison group of adults who took part in an 8-week training program (Figure 6.5; Ekblom & Goldbarg, 1971). Although the latter had no change in their RPE/HR ratio following training, the ratio for the children dropped from 0.82:10 to 0.55:10. Figure 6.6 summarizes the respective ratios in each of the acclimation

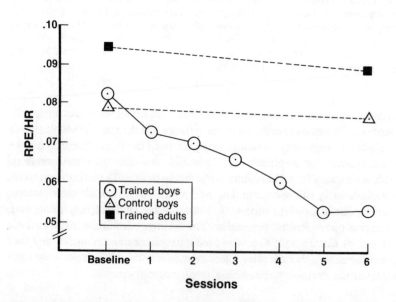

Figure 6.5 Changes in RPE/HR ratio (group means) during a 2-week aerobic program in 8- to 10-year-old boys compared with similar data from adults in an 8-week program (for protocols see text). *Note*. From "Relationship Between Perceptual and Physiological Changes During Heat Acclimatization in 8-10 Year-Old Boys" by O. Bar-Or and O. Inbar. In *Frontiers of Activity and Child Health* (p. 212) by H. Lavallée and R.J. Shephard (Eds.), 1977, Québec: Editions du Péli-can. Copyright 1977 by Editions du Pélican. Adapted by permission. Data for adults taken from "The Influence of Training and Other Factors on the Subjective Rating of Physical Exertion" by B. Ekblom and A.N. Goldbarg, 1971, *Acta Physiologica Scandinavica*, **83**, pp. 399-406.

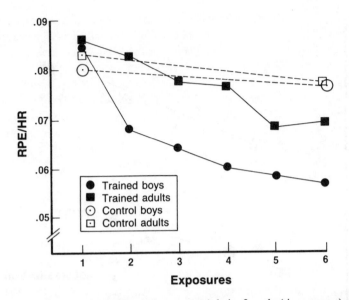

Figure 6.6 Changes in RPE/HR ratio (group means) during 2 weeks (six exposures) of acclimation to exercise in the heat in 8- to 10-year-old boys ($N = 9$) and in 20- to 23-year-old men ($N = 9$) compared with children and adults in control groups (for protocols see text). *Note*. From "Climate and the Exercising Child—A Review" by O. Bar-Or, 1980, *International Journal of Sports Medicine*, 1, p. 58. Copyright 1980. Reprinted by permission of Georg Thieme Verlag, Stuttgart.

sessions. Both acclimation groups had a gradual decline in the RPE/HR ratio, but it was significantly faster in the children. Child and adult controls had no change in RPE/HR.

A well-documented effect of aerobic training and, particularly, of acclimation to heat is a reduction in body core temperature during any given submaximal task. As expected, rectal temperature of the children in the study by Bar-Or and Inbar (1977) decreased by the end of the 2-week program. However, as shown in Figure 6.7, the reduction in RPE was above and beyond that expected from mere changes in core temperature. It was concluded that children's perceptual changes outpaced the reduction in physiologic strain during training and heat acclimation. The practical implication is that, when exposed to a heat wave (or when traveling to a warm climatic zone), children may be losing fast the restraining effect of subjective heat strain. Unless instructed to moderate their exercise intensity, such children may be at an excessive risk for heat-related illness.

RPE IN PRESCRIPTION

As early as 1970, Borg indicated that perceived exertion could be used, in analogy to monitoring of heart rate, in prescribing appropriate exercise intensities. This approach has been subsequently attempted in various studies with

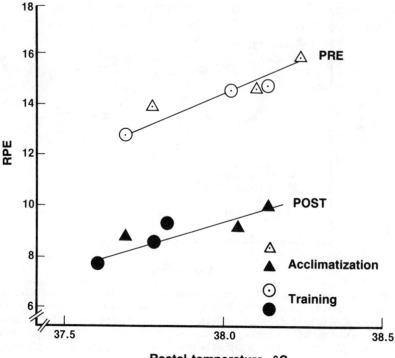

Figure 6.7 Relationship between RPE and rectal temperature (group means) in 8- to 10-year-old boys, before and after a 2-week heat acclimation and a training program (for protocol see text). *Note*. From "Relationship Between Perceptual and Physiological Changes During Heat Acclimatization in 8- to 10-Year-Old Boys" by O. Bar-Or and O. Inbar. In *Frontiers of Activity and Child Health* (p. 210) by H. Lavallée and R.J. Shephard (Eds.), 1977, Québec: Editions du Pélican. Copyright 1977 by Editions du Pélican. Reprinted by permission.

adults. An example is the work by Van Der Burg and Ceci (1986). Subjects first performed a graded treadmill test, during which the RPE concept was introduced to them. They were then asked to select a treadmill and a track running task, each equivalent to RPE 13. Speed of running on both the treadmill and on the track did not differ from that measured during the graded exercise test at RPE 13. Heart rates were very similar between the treadmill run and the graded exercise test, but on the running track they were some 20 beat $\cdot$ min^{-1} higher.

The possible use of RPE for exercise prescription with children has only recently been investigated (Ward & Bar-Or, 1987). Twenty mildly to moderately obese, 9- to 15-year-old girls and boys took part. After having been taught the RPE scale in two earlier cycle ergometry sessions, they were prescribed four different RPE levels (7, 10, 13, and 16) and asked to select the respective mechanical resistance, while pedaling at 50 rpm. On a separate day, they were asked to perform four 400-m walking/running tasks, as prescribed by the same RPE numbers. One finding was that these children were able to discriminate among the four cycling tasks (as based on the HR and the selected mechanical power) and, to a lesser extent, among the track tasks (based on HR and walking/ running velocities). However, as seen in Figure 6.8, their HR in the low-intensity cycling tasks was higher than expected. It was close to that expected at RPE 13, but too low at RPE 16. Thus it seems that, for prescribed cycling

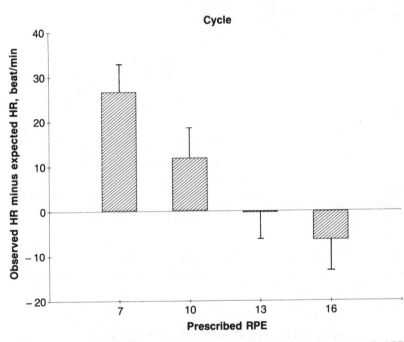

Figure 6.8 Accuracy of matching heart rate (means) and choice of intensity to prescribed RPE for 9- to 15-year-old obese children (vertical lines denote 1 SEM).

tasks, these children selected a too narrow range of intensities. As shown in Figure 6.9, they invariably—and at all prescribed tasks—exaggerated in their selection of walking/running intensities. Fourteen of the 20 children exercised on the track close to their maximal HR at each of the RPE prescription levels, including RPE 7.

Based on this study, one might conclude that children are less capable than adults of benefiting from the RPE prescription approach. This study, however, cannot be taken as definitive in this field. Additional work must be done with a more sophisticated teaching of the RPE concept and possibly with some anchoring technique that will imprint upon the child a more realistic range of exercise intensities. Preliminary information from the Children's Exercise

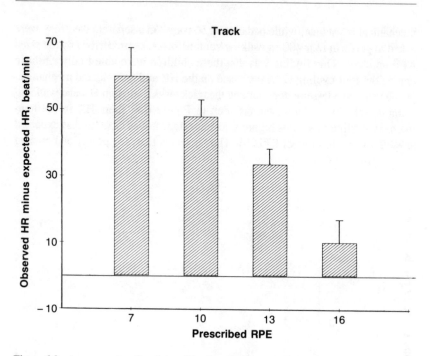

Figure 6.9 Accuracy of performing walking/running tasks on the track, as prescribed by RPE (variables, subjects, and notation are as in Figure 6.8).

and Nutrition Centre suggests that a simple feedback to the child about his or her success in selecting a walking/running speed improves the accuracy of selection in subsequent tasks.

CHALLENGES FOR FUTURE RESEARCH

Further research is indicated on RPE in children. Such research may not yield information on basic psychophysical phenomena, or on the mechanisms of exercise perception, but studies with children may help generate information that cannot be obtained by studying adults only. The following list of future research topics reflects the bias and interest of the authors and is not meant to be comprehensive.

- What is the *youngest age* at which a child can be expected to rate her or his perceived exertion reliably and with validity? A related question is whether it is the *chronological, biological, or mental age* that matters.
- Would young children rate better if a scale were constructed for them that, instead of numbers, has an *alternative notation* (e.g., pictures, line ranges, or colors)?

- Would *differential rating* (i.e., rating of leg effort vs. chest effort vs. total effort) *in healthy children* differ from that of adults? This may be the case because, compared with their maximal aerobic power, children's muscle strength and anaerobic power seem to be less developed.
- Likewise, one should assess the *differential rating in patients with pediatric diseases* that affect preferentially the musculoskeletal system (e.g., cerebral palsy, muscular dystrophy) or the oxygen transport system (e.g., cyanotic heart defect, cystic fibrosis).
- Development is needed of *methods for teaching and reinforcing the RPE concept for its use in exercise prescription.* Such methods are, most likely, different from those found useful with adults.

ACKNOWLEDGMENTS

The authors are indebted to staff members from the Children's Exercise and Nutrition Centre for their devoted help in data collection and analysis. Special thanks go to Michael Browne, Leslie McGillies, and Sherry Reed.

REFERENCES

Arstila, M., Antila, K., Wendelin, H., Vuori, I., & Välimäki, I. (1977). The effect of age and sex on the perception of exertion during an exercise test with a linear increase in heart rate. In G. Borg (Ed.), *Physical work and effort* (pp. 217-221). Oxford: Pergamon.

Bar-Or, O. (1977). Age-related changes in exercise perception. In G. Borg (Ed). *Physical work and effort* (pp. 255-266). Oxford: Pergamon.

Bar-Or, O. (1980). Climate and the exercising child—a review. *International Journal of Sports Medicine,* **1,** 53-65.

Bar-Or, O. (1983). *Pediatric sports medicine for the practitioner.* New York: Springer-Verlag.

Bar-Or, O., & Inbar, O. (1977). Relationship between perceptual and physiological changes during heat acclimatization in 8-10 year old boys. In H. Lavallée & R.J. Shephard (Eds.), *Frontiers of activity and child health* (pp. 205-214). Québec: Editions du Pélican.

Bar-Or, O., & Reed, S.L. (1986). Rating of perceived exertion of adolescents with neuromuscular disease. In G. Borg & D. Ottoson (Eds.), *The perception of exertion in physical work* (pp. 137-148). Basingstoke, England: Macmillan.

Bar-Or, O., Skinner, J.S., Buskirk, E.R., & Borg, G. (1972). Physiological and perceptual indicators of physical stress in 41- to 60-year-old men who vary in conditioning level and in body fat. *Medicine and Science in Sports,* **4,** 96-100.

Birk, T., Gavron, S., Ross, J., Hackett, K., Boullard, K., Olson, R., & Gosling, R. (1983, April). *Relationship of perceived exertion and heart rate response during exercise testing in wheelchair users.* Paper presented at the annual convention of the American Alliance for Health, Physical Education, Recreation and Dance, Minneapolis, MN.

Bjuro, T., Fugl-Meyer, A.R., Grimby, G., Hook, O., & Lundgren, B. (1975). Ergonomic studies of standardized domestic work in patients with neuromuscular handicap. *Scandinavian Journal of Rehabilitation Medicine, 7,* 106-113.

Borg, G. (1962). *Physical performance and perceived exertion.* Lund, Sweden: Gleerup.

Borg, G. (1970). Perceived exertion as an indicator of somatic stress. *Scandinavian Journal of Rehabilitation Medicine, 2-3,* 92-98.

Borg, G. (1977). *Physical work and effort.* Oxford: Pergamon.

Borg, G. (1982). Psychophysical bases of perceived exertion. *Medicine and Science in Sports and Exercise, 14,* 377-381.

Cafarelli, E. (1982). Peripheral contributions to the perception of effort. *Medicine and Science in Sports and Exercise, 14,* 382-389.

Carton, R.L., & Rhodes, E.C. (1985). A critical review of the literature on rating scales for perceived exertion. *Sports Medicine, 2,* 198-222.

Dally, P. (1969). *Anorexia nervosa.* London: Heinemann Medical Books.

Davies, C.T.M., Fohlin, L., & Thorén, C. (1980). Perception of exertion in anorexia nervosa patients. In K. Berg & B.O. Eriksson (Eds.), *Children and exercise* (Vol. 9, pp. 327-332). Baltimore: University Park Press.

Docktor, R., & Sharkey, B. (1971). Note on some physiological and subjective reactions to exercise and training. *Perceptual and Motor Skills, 32,* 233-234.

Ekblom, B., & Goldbarg, A.N. (1971). The influence of training and other factors on the subjective rating of physical exertion. *Acta Physiologica Scandinavica, 83,* 399-406.

Eriksson, B.O., Karlsson, J., & Saltin, B. (1971). Muscle metabolites during exercise in pubertal boys. *Acta Paediatrica Scandinavica,* (Suppl. 217), 154-157.

Kahle, C.J., Ulmer, H.V., & Rummel, L. (1977). The reproducibility of Borg's RPE-Scale of female pupils from 7 to 11 years of age (Abstract). *Pflügers Archiv: European Journal of Physiology,* (Suppl. 368), R26.

Kilbom, Å. (1971). Physical training in women. *Scandinavian Journal of Clinical and Laboratory Investigation, 28*(Suppl. 119), 1-34.

Komi, P.V., & Karppi, S.-L. (1977). Genetic and environmental variation in perceived exertion and heart rate during bicycle ergometer work. In G. Borg (Ed.), *Physical work and effort* (pp. 91-99). Oxford: Pergamon.

Miyashita, M., Onodera, K., & Tabata, I. (1986). How Borg's scale has been applied to Japanese. In G. Borg & D. Ottoson (Eds.), *The perception of exertion in physical work* (pp. 27-34). Basingstoke, England: Macmillan.

Nordemar, R., Edstrom, L., & Ekblom, B. (1976). Changes in muscle fibre size and physical performance in patients with rheumatoid arthritis after short-term physical training. *Scandinavian Journal of Rheumatology, 5,* 70-76.

Pandolf, K.B. (1982). Advances in the study and application of perceived exertion. *Exercise and Sort Sciences Reviews, 11,* 118-158.

Pandolf, K.B., Burse, R.L., & Goldman, R.F. (1975). Differential ratings of perceived exertion during physical conditioning for older individuals using leg-weight loading. *Perceptual and Motor Skills, 40,* 563-574.

Robertson, R.J. (1982). Central signals of perceived exertion during dynamic exercise. *Medicine and Science in Sports and Exercise, 14,* 390-396.

Rutenfranz, J., Klimt, F., Ilmarinen, J., & Kylian, H. (1977). Blood lactate concentration during triangular and stepwise loading on the bicycle ergometer. In H. Lavallée & R.J. Shephard (Eds.), *Frontiers of activity and child health* (pp. 179-187). Québec: Editions du Pélican.

Sargeant, A.J., & Davies, C.T.M. (1977). Perceived exertion of dynamic exercise in normal subjects and patients following leg injury. In G. Borg (Ed.), *Physical work and effort* (pp. 345-355). Oxford: Pergamon.

Skinner, J.S., Borg, G.A.V., & Buskirk, E.R. (1969). Physiological and perceptual reaction to exertion of young men differing in activity and body size. In B.D. Franks (Ed.), *Exercise and fitness* (pp. 53-66). Chicago: Athletic Institute.

Skinner, J.S., Hustler, R., Bergsteinová, V., & Buskirk, E.R. (1973a). Perception of effort during different types of exercise and under different environmental conditions. *Medicine and Science in Sports, 5,* 110-115.

Skinner, J.S., Hustler, R., Bergsteinová, V., & Buskirk, E.R. (1973b). The validity and reliability of a rating scale of perceived exertion. *Medicine and Science in Sports, 5,* 94-96.

Stamford, B.A. (1976). Validity and reliability of subjective ratings of perceived exertion during work. *Ergonomics, 1,* 53-60.

Ulmer, H.-V., Janz, U., & Lollgen, H. (1977). Aspects of the validity of Borg's scale. Is it measuring stress or strain? In G. Borg (Ed.), *Physical work and effort* (pp. 181-196). Oxford: Pergamon.

Van der Burg, M., & Ceci, R. (1986). A comparison of a psychophysical estimation and a production method in a laboratory and a field condition. In G. Borg & D. Ottosen (Eds.), *The perception of exertion in physical work* (pp. 35-46). Basingstoke, England: Macmillan.

Van Huss, W.D., Stephens, K.E., Vogel, P., Anderson, D., Kurowski, T.,

Janes, J.A., & Fitzgerald, C. (1986). Physiological and perceptual responses of elite age group distance runners during progressive intermittent work to exhaustion. *The 1984 Olympic Scientific Congress Proceedings,* **10**, 239-256.

Ward, D.S., & Bar-Or, O. (1987). Usefulness of RPE scale for exercise prescription with obese youth (Abstract). *Medicine and Science in Sports and Exercise,* **19**, S15.

Ward, D.S., & Bar-Or, O. (in press). Use of the Borg scale for exercise prescription with obese youth. *Canadian Journal of Sport Sciences.*

Ward, D.S., Blimkie, C.J.R., & Bar-Or, O. (1986). Rating of perceived exertion in obese adolescents (Abstract). *Medicine and Science in Sports and Exercise,* **18**, S72.

7

Iron Deficiency and Supplementation in the Young Endurance Athlete

Thomas W. Rowland
Baystate Medical Center, Springfield, Massachusetts

The essential role of iron in the maintenance of good health has been appreciated since antiquity. Patients complaining of weakness were treated by the ancient Greeks with iron, administered as water in which swords had been allowed to rust. In the late seventeenth century, Sydenham prescribed "iron or steel filings steeped in cold Rhenish wine—to the worn out or languid it gives a spur or fillip whereby the animal spirits which lay prostrate and sunken under their own weight are raised and excited" (Herbert, 1965, p. 1394). More contemporary physicians have added little to this therapeutic approach, although the vehicle for administration of iron may have changed.

With the subsequent understanding of the key role of iron in the formation of hemoglobin (Hb), the salutary effects of iron treatment on symptoms of fatigue and lethargy became more easily explained. Iron deficiency of sufficient degree to inhibit Hb synthesis and decrease red blood cell production can be expected to reduce oxygen transport to tissues, a particular detriment during endurance physical exercise when contracting muscle oxygen demands increase dramatically. This concept of iron deficiency anemia impairing exercise performance by limiting oxygen delivery has been repeatedly supported by studies of anemic animals, healthy human volunteers, and both adults and children in underdeveloped nations (Cook & Lynch, 1986; Davies, 1974; Greisen, 1986; Woodson, 1984; Wranne & Woodson, 1973). Furthermore, experimental evidence suggests that exercise performance may be increased in athletes when Hb concentrations are raised above normal by transfusion of autologous red blood cells (Buick, Gledhill, Froese, Spriet, & Meyers, 1980).

Recent data indicate that iron deficiency in the absence of anemia (Hb < 12 g • dL^{-1} in females and < 13 g • dL^{-1} in males) may also impair endurance exercise capacity by interfering with intracellular aerobic metabolism (Finch et al., 1976; Rowland, Deisroth, Green, & Kelleher, 1987). The implications of nonanemic iron deficiency may be significant, because (a) this condition appears to be common in endurance athletes, particularly distance runners; and (b) iron deficiency is easily identified and treated with oral iron supplementation.

Although attention to iron deficiency has been focused principally on adult athletes, the potential influence of iron depletion on sports performance is clearly a pediatric concern as well. Iron deficiency is of particular importance to adolescent athletes who are experiencing increasing body iron requirements during periods of rapid growth. In addition, the consequences of iron depletion may not be limited solely to exercise performance. Disturbances of growth, immune function, gastrointestinal activity, and behavior have all been linked to iron deficiency during the pediatric years (Oski, 1979).

This review describes the biochemical basis for nonanemic iron deficiency and its influence on aerobic metabolism, examines available information regarding the impact of this condition on exercise in humans and animals, and relates these findings to possible options for counseling adolescent athletes regarding iron supplementation.

BODY IRON STORES, SERUM FERRITIN, AND AEROBIC METABOLISM

Although the total body iron content is small (3.5-4.0 g in the average adult male), ferrous compounds are essential for life. Because these substances provide key links in oxygen transport (Hb) and intracellular oxygen metabolism (myoglobin, cytochromes), adequate iron stores are critical for meeting the aerobic demands of endurance exercise. Approximately two-thirds of body iron is used in the synthesis of Hb, whereas only 5% contributes to the formation or function of myoglobin, cytochromes, cytochrome oxidase, succinic dehydrogenase, and xanthine oxidase (Herbert, 1965; Latner, 1975). These latter

substances all play important roles in intracellular oxidation; it would therefore be expected that depletion of body iron stores might limit exercise performance by impaired intracellular aerobic metabolism as well as by diminished
oxygen transport from iron deficiency anemia (Clement & Sawchuck, 1984;
Oski, 1979). The remaining 20%-30% of body iron is stored in the liver and
reticuloendothelial system as ferritin, an iron-protein complex, or hemosiderin
(Figure 7.1). The concentration of ferritin in serum is a direct reflection of
tissue ferritin and serves as a useful marker of body iron stores (Jacobs &
Worwood, 1975).

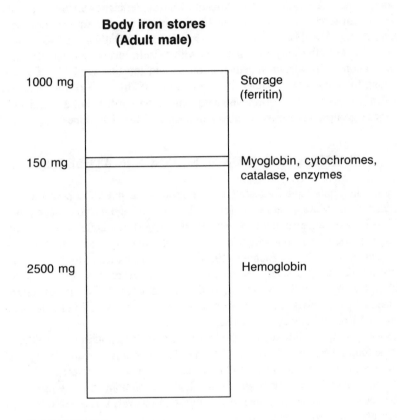

**Body iron stores
(Adult male)**

1000 mg — Storage (ferritin)

150 mg — Myoglobin, cytochromes, catalase, enzymes

2500 mg — Hemoglobin

Total 3500 mg

Figure 7.1 Distribution of body iron content in the normal adult male.

Deficiency of body iron may result from either inadequate oral intake or
excessive loss through hemorrhage, stools, urine, or sweat. Body ferritin stores
fall during the early stages of iron depletion without influencing normal Hb
synthesis (Clement & Sawchuck, 1984). Mild degrees of iron deficiency are

therefore typified by reduced serum ferritin levels but normal Hb concentrations. In this stage of nonanemic iron deficiency, concentrations of intracellular iron-dependent factors (e.g., myoglobin, cytochromes) may be reduced, creating the potential for impairment of aerobic metabolism in the absence of diminished Hb concentration (Finch et al., 1976). Disturbances of Hb synthesis with overt anemia and reduced arterial oxygen content are thus a late manifestation of progressive iron deficiency, marked by reduced serum concentrations of both ferritin and Hb.

Estimates of normal ferritin values have been derived by population studies as well as phlebotomy, marrow aspiration, and iron absorption measurements (Cook, Finch, & Smith, 1976). Patients with iron deficiency anemia typically have serum ferritin levels less than 12 ng • mL^{-1}, a value equivalent to less than 100 mg of total storage iron (Siimes, Addiego, & Dallman, 1974). Siimes et al. (1974) found only four subjects with ferritin levels less than 10 ng • mL^{-1} among 118 normal nonanemic males and females aged 11–15 years. Among the adolescents studied by Cook et al. (1976), 12% of the boys and 25% of the girls had ferritin levels less than 12 ng • mL^{-1}, but 2% and 11% of these groups, respectively, also demonstrated low Hb values.

FREQUENCY OF IRON DEFICIENCY IN ATHLETES

Reports in adults have indicated an increased frequency of nonanemic iron deficiency in endurance athletes (Table 7.1). Although these studies have usually involved distance runners, recent reports suggest that athletes in a variety of sports, including non-weight-bearing events, may also be at high risk of iron depletion (Selby & Eichner, 1986). Some data indicate, moreover, that ferritin levels progressively fall during the course of training (Frederickson, Puhl, & Runyan, 1983; Rowland, Black, & Kelleher, 1987). In all reports female athletes consistently demonstrate lower ferritin levels and higher incidence of iron deficiency compared to males.

Bone marrow studies support the reality of iron depletion in these athletes. Of the total 20 runners studied by Wishnitzer, Vorst, and Berrebi (1983), and Ehn, Carlmark, and Hoglund (1980), 11 demonstrated a complete absence of storage iron and 8 had markedly diminished iron on bone marrow aspirates. Hb concentrations were normal in all subjects; however, serum ferritin levels were not obtained in either study.

When adolescent distance runners are examined, a similar high frequency of iron deficiency is observed (Table 7.2). Rowland et al. (1987) studied high school male and female cross-country runners with measurement of serum ferritin, Hb, and red cell indexes during an 11-week competitive season. Eight of 20 females (40%) and one male of 30 (3%) had iron deficiency (serum ferritin < 12 ng • mL^{-1}) without anemia at the beginning of the season. By the end of the study period, four additional males and another female became iron depleted, for an overall incidence of 17% of males and 45% of females. These

Table 7.1 Iron Deficiency in Adult Athletes

Authors	Subjects	Sex	Findings
Parr et al. (1984)	Collegiate track, softball, field hockey	F	Mean ferritin 16.8 ng · mL^{-1} compared to 25.9 ng · mL^{-1} in controls.
Clement & Asmundson (1982)	College distance runners	M/F	82% of females, 29% of males had ferritin < 25 ng · mL^{-1}.
Lampe et al. (1986)	Marathon runners	M/F	32% of females, 7% of males had ferritin < 20 ng · mL^{-1}.
Selby & Eichner (1986)	Master's and collegiate swimmers	M/F	12% of males, 50% of females had ferritin < 15 ng · mL^{-1}.
Crowell et al. (1985)	Endurance trained	M	Mean ferritin 63 ng · mL^{-1} compared to 92 ng · mL^{-1} in controls.
Colt & Heyman (1984)	Nonelite competitive runners	F	Mean ferritin 17.8 ng · mL^{-1}; controls 69.6 ng · mL^{-1}.
		M	Mean ferritin 61.4 ng · mL^{-1}; controls 98.4 ng · mL^{-1}.
Dufaux et al. (1981)	Distance runners	M	Significantly lower ferritin levels than controls or cyclists.
Dickson et al. (1982)	Ultramarathon runners	M	14% ferritin < 30 ng · mL^{-1}.
	Trained swimmers	M	None had ferritin < 30 ng · mL^{-1}.
Haymes et al. (1986)	Olympic cross-country skiers	F	Progressive fall in ferritin levels with training.

values represent a conservative estimate, because only 31 of the 50 runners were evaluated throughout the entire season. Of the 26 runners who were studied during the season, ferritin levels declined in all 9 females and in 14 of 17 males. No subject developed evidence of disturbed red blood cell production.

Nickerson and Tripp (1983) screened 18 female high school cross-country runners for iron deficiency after 1 month of regular training. Of those with normal Hb concentrations, 9 of 18 had serum ferritin values less than 10 ng • mL^{-1}. If the criterion for iron deficiency was raised to 20 ng • mL^{-1}, two-thirds (12/18) demonstrated nonanemic iron deficiency. In a second study of adolescent runners, Nickerson, Holubets, Tripp, and Pierce (1985) described serum ferritin levels of less than 20 ng • mL^{-1} in 8 of 20 subjects (40%) by the end of a competitive season.

Fredrickson et al. (1983) evaluated eight female runners through a season for hematologic evidence of impaired red blood cell formation. Progressive fall in serum iron and percent transferrin saturation occurred with increase in free erythrocyte protoporphyrin and total iron-binding capacity. These values, which are all indicative of increasingly significant iron deficiency, returned toward normal in the detraining period after the end of the season.

Based on blood ferritin and Hb levels, the incidence of nonanemic iron deficiency in adolescent runners therefore appears to be at least as high as that previously described in adult endurance athletes. The marked predilection for females and the pattern of progressive iron depletion with training also mimic characteristics of iron deficiency observed in older athletes.

THE ETIOLOGY OF IRON DEFICIENCY IN ATHLETES

Why iron deficiency should be so prevalent in endurance athletes remains unclear. Iron depletion signifies an imbalance between nutritive intake and body losses, and regular physical activity may stimulate more than one mechanism that leads to a chronic drain of body iron stores. As noted, theories regarding the etiology of iron deficiency in athletes must consider (a) the consistently higher incidence of iron depletion in females, (b) the progressive severity of hypoferritinemia that occurs during the course of training, and (c) increasing evidence that iron deficiency is not limited to athletes engaged in weight-bearing sports (e.g., running).

Diet. Normally, nutritional requirements for iron are not high (Latner, 1975). Daily body iron losses in the adult male, which must be replenished in the diet, amount to less than 1.0 mg (about 0.03% of total stores). Typical losses from menstrual bleeding amount to an additional 0.05-0.08 mg • day^{-1}. During adolescence, the marked increase in iron needs to sustain a rapidly enlarging hemoglobin mass causes the iron requirement to be greater than at any other time in life (approximately 1.5 times that of adult age; Herbert, 1965).

Table 7.2 Iron Deficiency in Adolescent Athletes

Authors	Subjects	Sex	Findings
Rowland, Black, et al. (1987)	Cross-country runners	M/F	45% of females, 17% of males had ferritin < 12 ng $\cdot$ mL^{-1}.
Nickerson & Tripp (1983)	Cross-country runners	F	67% had ferritin < 20 ng $\cdot$ mL^{-1}.
Nickerson et al. (1985)	Cross-country runners	F	40% had ferritin < 20 ng $\cdot$ mL^{-1}.
Frederickson et al. (1983)	Cross-country runners	F	Decreasing serum iron in all eight subjects with training.

Because only approximately 10% of nutritional iron is absorbed in the gastrointestinal tract, daily iron ingestion must equal tenfold the daily requirement to match these losses and increased demands. Iron intake less than 10-15 mg in the adolescent male and 15-25 mg in the adolescent female per day might therefore be expected to eventuate in signs of iron deficiency.

Foods rich in iron, including liver, lima beans, shellfish, and green vegetables, are not notably tempting to teenagers, and diets of adolescents are, therefore, often low in iron content (Wurtman, 1981). Runners consume diets high in complex carbohydrates and typically avoid red meat (a rich source of readily absorbed heme iron), creating an even greater chance for dietary iron inadequacy. A dietary recall questionnaire administered by Frederickson et al. (1983) to eight high school female cross-country runners indicated an average daily iron intake of only 14.7 mg. Among the 35 female high school runners studied by Nickerson et al. (1985), the mean daily iron intake was approximately 10 mg, with 83% taking in less than 14 mg. Forty percent of the subjects had ferritin levels less than 20 ng $\cdot$ mL^{-1}. Similar findings have been observed in adult runners. Clement and Asmundson (1982) evaluated diets of collegiate distance runners using 7-day individual dietary surveys. The mean daily iron intake in females was 12.5 mg, and almost 91% ingested less than 14 mg. Iron intake in the men was usually adequate, with a mean of 18.5 mg $\cdot$ day^{-1}. As indicated previously, 82% of the women and 29% of the men had ferritin levels less than 25 ng $\cdot$ mL^{-1}. Snyder, Dvorak, and Roepke (1987) demonstrated lower mean ferritin levels in a group of nine vegetarian middle-aged female runners (7.4) compared to those consuming red meat (19.8).

The typical iron-poor diets of endurance athletes are, therefore, a major risk factor for iron deficiency and may contribute significantly to their low ferritin levels.

Hemolysis. Hemolysis, or the premature breakdown of red blood cells, has long been suspected to play a role in iron deficiency in runners because of the repetitive trauma to the capillaries of the feet from the impacts incurred during training and competition. Recent data support the increased frequency of hemolysis in runners, but the role of red cell breakdown in iron deficiency is controversial (Carlson & Mawdsley, 1986; Martin, Vroon, May, & Pilbeam, 1986; Steenkamp, Fuller, Graves, Noakes, & Jacobs, 1986).

Iron released with hemolysis binds to haptoglobin in the blood; a fall in the concentration of free haptoglobin therefore serves as a useful measure of the degree of hemolysis. The process of hemolysis itself does not typically lead to iron deficiency, because the released iron is recycled by the body to be used in the formation of new red blood cells. When the rate of hemolysis is high, however, the freed iron exceeds the binding capacity of haptoglobin and is cleared from plasma into the urine, resulting in body iron loss as hemoglobinuria.

Magnusson, Hallberg, Rossander, and Swolin (1984a) demonstrated low haptoglobin values in 9 of 12 adult male runners but no iron loss in the urine, and Dressendorfer, Wade, and Amsterdam (1981) showed that frank hemoglobinuria was rare even during several days of road racing. Other authors, however, demonstrated hemoglobinuria after vigorous exercise (Buckle & Cantab, 1965; Gilligan, Altshule, & Katersky, 1943). Therefore, whereas reduced haptoglobin levels are not uncommon in competitive runners (Clement & Sawchuck, 1984), it is unclear whether this process does, in fact, contribute significantly to iron loss.

The explanation for hemolysis in these athletes is also uncertain. The runners have demonstrated less evidence of hemolysis when wearing air-cushioned shoes compared to conventional firm-soled shoes (Falsetti, Burke, Feld, Frederick, & Ratering, 1983). However, evidence of hemolysis in participants in non-weight-bearing sports indicates that mechanical trauma to the feet is not the only factor involved. Selby and Eichner (1986) demonstrated low haptoglobin levels in 26% of master's and collegiate swimmers and suggested that hemolysis might result from vigorous contracting muscles or changes in erythrocyte and plasma osmolality. Others have proposed that trauma from the increased circulatory rate, rise in body temperature (Clement & Sawchuck, 1984), or release of adrenalin (Carlson & Mawdsley, 1986) could serve as other mechanisms responsible for exercise-induced hemolysis.

Hemorrhage. Gastrointestinal bleeding is a well-recognized phenomenon in competitive runners, particularly following distance races. McMahon, Ryan, Larson, and Fisher (1984) described 7 of 32 runners with positive stool tests for blood after a marathon, and Lampe, Ellefson, Slavin, Schwartz, and Apple (1987) reported a similar incidence in female marathon competitors. Peak losses in the latter study were substantial, amounting to 4.7 mL (approximately 3 mg of iron) per day. Twenty-nine percent of the runners reported by Stewart, Ahlquist, and McGill (1984) lost at least 2 mg of iron daily in stools following a marathon race. Cantwell (1987) described two runners experiencing bloody diarrhea and abdominal pain with training and suggested gut ischemia as a cause, because 80% of normal gastrointestinal blood flow may be shunted away during exercise (Clausen, 1977).

Blood loss in the urine may also contribute to iron loss. Hematuria following running may result from hypoxia-induced glomerular permeability or bladder trauma (Alyea & Parish, 1958; Blacklock, 1977). Of the 50 male runners in the 1978 Boston Marathon studied by Siegel, Hennekens, Solomon, and VanBoeckel (1979), 9 demonstrated hematuria, which cleared by 48 hr.

Exaggerated menstrual blood loss is the most common cause of iron deficiency in adolescent and adult nonathletic females, and the predominance of hypoferritinemia in female runners clearly suggests menstruation as a contributing factor. Oligomenorrhea, however, is more common in highly competitive athletes, and the 35 high school cross-country runners studied by Nickerson et al. (1985) reported no excessive menstrual bleeding.

Other Losses. The concentration of iron in sweat is low (approximately

0.2 mg • L^{-1}) and losses are normally minimal by this route. With very heavy sweating during exercise, however, iron losses may approach 1 mg (Vellar, 1968). Ehn et al. (1980) used whole-body counting of radioactive labeled iron to demonstrate a more rapid elimination of body iron in distance runners. No evidence of bleeding, hemolysis, or hemoglobinuria was observed; increased loss of iron in sweat was therefore proposed as a possible mechanism. Rhabdomyolysis, the breakdown of muscle cells, may occur with strenuous exercise, resulting in myoglobin loss in the urine; however, myoglobinuria appears to be unusual in runners (Boileau, Fuchs, & Barry, 1980).

THE INFLUENCE OF NONANEMIC IRON DEFICIENCY ON EXERCISE PERFORMANCE

Studies on animals indicate that nonanemic iron deficiency impairs exercise performance by affecting the function of intracellular, iron-dependent factors important in aerobic metabolism. Limited human experiments, however, have produced conflicting results.

In their classic study in rats, Finch et al. (1976) demonstrated a clear-cut influence of iron depletion on treadmill running performance in nonanemic animals. Four groups of rats were maintained throughout the study at identical Hb concentrations by intermittent removal and addition of blood through an intravascular catheter. The animals in Group A were fed an iron-deficient diet for 4 weeks prior to the exercise testing period. The Group B rats consumed a normal diet. Animals in Group C were maintained on the iron-deficient diet but were also given an iron supplement. Group D rats ate the iron-deficient diet but were started on oral iron at the beginning of the testing period.

During treadmill testing the rats fed the iron-deficient diet could run for only 4 min, whereas those consuming either a normal diet or on iron-deficient diet with iron supplementation endured for 16 to 20 min (Figure 7.2). The rats fed the iron-deficient diet and then started on iron at the beginning of exercise testing could only run for 4 min initially, but after 1 day of iron treatment this increased to 10 min; endurance time progressively increased thereafter so that by 3 days the exercise performance was the same as those fed normal diets. In the iron-deficient rats the muscle concentration of cytochrome pigments and myoglobin, as well as activities of succinic dehydrogenase and alpha-glycerophosphate, were diminished. Only the rate of phosphorylation with alpha-glycerophosphate increased with iron therapy, however, suggesting this metabolic step was most influenced by iron deficiency. These findings clearly indicated that iron deficiency in animals with normal Hb concentrations can limit exercise capacity.

Davies, Maguire, Brooks, Dallman and Packer (1982) examined muscle oxidative function and treadmill performance in rats made severely iron deficient and anemic by a low-iron diet. When the animals were given supplementary

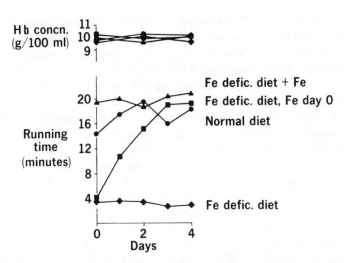

Figure 7.2 Response of treadmill running time in rats with iron treatment. *Note.* Data from Finch et al., 1976. Figure from "The Nonhematologic Manifestations of Iron Deficiency" by F.A. Oski, 1976, *American Journal of Diseases of Children, 133*, p. 320. Copyright 1976 by American Journal of Diseases of Children. Reprinted by permission.

iron, the Hb concentration increased substantially within 3 days, paralleling the rise in maximum oxygen consumption ($\dot{V}O_2$max) during treadmill running. No improvements were observed until the 5th day, however, in mitochondrial content of muscle, muscle oxidative capacity, or endurance times. They concluded that $\dot{V}O_2$ was not limited by muscle oxidative capacity and that endurance time was restricted by muscle oxidative capacity rather than oxygen supply.

Other studies have demonstrated the dissociation of $\dot{V}O_2$max and endurance time in rats and suggest separate roles of iron in red blood cell production and cellular aerobic metabolism in influencing limits to exercise. Davies, Donovan, Refino, Brooks, and Packer (1984) showed that partial transfusion to anemic, iron-deficient animals improved $\dot{V}O_2$max but had no effect on endurance time. Perkkio, Jansson, Brooks, Refino, and Dallman (1985) demonstrated a decrease in $\dot{V}O_2$max in rats only when Hb concentrations fell below $7 \text{ g} \cdot dL^{-1}$. Treadmill endurance time, however, fell abruptly when Hb declined to $8-10$ $\text{g} \cdot dL^{-1}$, a point where $\dot{V}O_2$ was virtually unchanged. These findings suggest that, although iron deficiency anemia mainly impairs $\dot{V}O_2$max, muscle iron depletion affects endurance time by interfering with intracellular aerobic metabolism. They further imply that nonanemic iron deficiency in humans might affect running endurance time without altering $\dot{V}O_2$max.

The findings of Rowland, Deisroth, Green, and Kelleher (1987) after iron treatment of female high school runners with nonanemic iron deficiency support this concept. Fourteen cross-country runners with initial ferritin levels of less than 20 ng • mL⁻¹ and normal Hb values were studied with serial determinations of hematologic and treadmill running parameters during a competitive season. After a 4-week control period, the runners were treated for 1 month with either ferrous sulfate (975 mg • day⁻¹) or placebo in a double-blind fashion. Ferritin levels rose during iron treatment from a mean of 8.7 to 26.6 ng • mL⁻¹, whereas they fell in the placebo group to a mean of 8.6 ng • mL⁻¹ by the end of the season. Six of seven subjects improved treadmill endurance time while being treated with iron (range 0.03 to 1.92 min), whereas performance fell in all seven controls (range −0.07 to −1.30 min; Figure 7.3). The increased duration of exercise time in the treated group was not significantly different from that indicated by training alone during the first part of the season. This indicates that iron supplementation in a nondeficient subject will not improve endurance performance. A direct relationship was observed between individual ferritin levels at the end of the season and change in treadmill endurance time during treatment. No significant differences in maximal or submaximal V̇O₂, ventilation, or heart rate were demonstrated between the two groups.

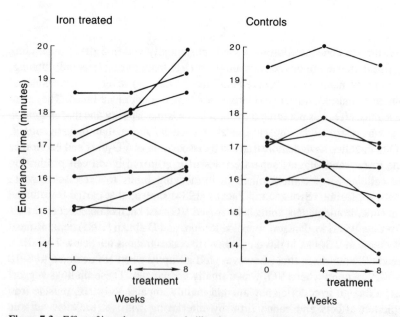

Figure 7.3 Effect of iron therapy on treadmill endurance time in female high school cross country runners treated between weeks four and eight of competitive season (left) versus controls. *Note.* From "The Effect of Iron Therapy on the Exercise Capacity of Non-Anemic Iron Deficient Adolescent Runners" by T.W. Rowland, M.B. Deisroth, G.M. Green, and J.F. Kelleher, 1988, *American Journal of Diseases of Children*, **142**, pp. 165-169. Copyright 1988 by the American Journal of Diseases of Children. Reprinted by permission.

Other less direct studies have also suggested the influence of nonanemic iron deficiency in impairing exercise performance. Schoene et al. (1983) reported a decline in maximal exercise lactate concentrations after iron treatment in female college endurance athletes with initial low ferritin levels but normal Hb concentrations; however, no significant difference in maximum exercise performance was observed after iron therapy. Ohira et al. (1979) described improved work capacity and lower submaximal heart rates after treating iron deficient anemic subjects that could not be fully explained by increases in Hb. Ericsson (1970) reported that nonanemic elderly adults improved their physical work capacity (cycle ergometry) after treatment with oral iron.

However, Celsing, Blomstrand, Werner, Pihlstedt, and Ekblom (1986) could not demonstrate impaired treadmill endurance times or $\dot{V}O_2$max in nonanemic adult males using an artificially induced iron deficiency protocol. Iron depletion and decreased Hb concentration were induced by repeated phlebotomy over a 9-week period. A state of nonanemic iron deficiency was then created by retransfusion of blood. Muscle biopsy analysis of glycolytic, oxidative, and iron-dependent enzymes indicated no significant activity changes during the control, anemic, or retransfusion stages of the study. Running times to exhaustion and $\dot{V}O_2$max fell after repeat phlebotomies, but after retransfusion to normal Hb values both of these parameters returned to normal (despite a mean ferritin level of 9.1 ng • mL^{-1}).

Matter et al. (1987) examined 11 adult female marathon runners with serum ferritin levels of less than 40 ng • mL^{-1} and normal Hb concentrations. No significant changes in maximum treadmill running time, $\dot{V}O_2$max, peak lactate levels, or anaerobic threshold were observed during treatment despite increases in serum ferritin levels. The average ferritin value of the subjects before treatment, however, was 30 ng • mL^{-1}, a level above that usually accepted as indicating iron depletion (Cook et al., 1976). As the authors emphasized, increasing ferritin levels within the normal range does not appear to enhance performance, which provides a possible explanation for failure of these runners to improve endurance with iron therapy.

The foregoing discussion has assumed that low ferritin levels in athletes represent true iron deficiency, a conclusion that is not without its detractors. Magnusson Hallberg, Rossander, and Swolin (1984b) have suggested that the formation of hemoglobin-haptoglobin complexes from hemolysis during training and competition shunts iron away from normal metabolic pathways that usually eventuate in ferritin deposition as storage iron (Figure 7.4). According to this view, reduced serum ferritin levels in athletes are thus not a true reflection of depletion of body iron stores. As such, hypoferritinemia without anemia does not represent a physiologic impairment and does not signal a need for iron therapy.

Magnusson et al. (1984b) based their argument on hematologic findings in a large group of adult male distance runners. Serum ferritin, haptoglobin, and bone marrow hemosiderin were reduced compared to controls, but even in

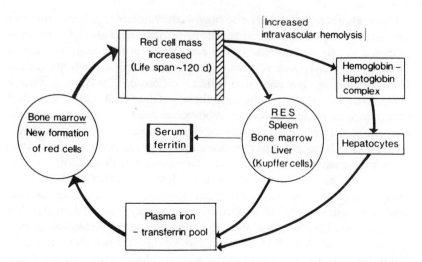

Figure 7.4 Proposed iron pathways in athletes. Increased hemolysis (right) shunts iron away from pathways that usually lead to ferritin deposition, resulting in low serum ferritin levels without true body iron depletion. *Note.* From "Iron Metabolism and 'Sports Anemia.' I and II" by B. Magnusson, L. Hallberg, L. Rossander, and B. Swolin, 1984, *Acta Medica Scandinavica*, **216**, p. 162. Copyright 1984 by Acta Medica Scandinavica and the authors. Reprinted by permission.

subjects with virtual absence of storage iron on bone marrow smears there was no evidence of impaired red blood cell production (i.e., normal bone marrow sideroblast count, red blood cell protoporphyrin values, mean corpuscular volume, and Hb concentrations). In another study (Magnusson, Hallberg, Rossander, & Swolin, 1984a), 22 iron parameters were compared in five runners with low serum ferritin (< 25 ng • mL^{-1}) or markedly decreased bone marrow hemosiderin, with seven having ferritin levels over 100, or abundant bone marrow hemosiderin. No differences in dietary iron intake, red blood cell volume, hemoglobin concentration, urinary iron loss, or mean corpuscular volume were observed between the two groups. When desferroxamine (an iron-chelating agent) was administered to both groups, urinary iron losses were 0.80 ($\pm$ 0.19) mg • day^{-1} in the iron-deficient group and 0.98 ($\pm$ 0.52) mg • day^{-1} in the nondeficient group, a statistically insignificant difference. The authors concluded that there was no rational basis for routine iron therapy in athletes.

The findings of Rowland et al. (1987) of impaired treadmill endurance times in high school runners with low ferritin levels appear to refute this argument. However, the fact that several runners in that study participated with ferritin levels as low as 3-4 ng • mL^{-1} with normal Hb and mean corpuscular volume values is puzzling. Because individuals with overt iron deficiency anemia have similar ferritin levels (Siimes et al., 1974), the explanation for lack of impaired Hb synthesis and red blood cell formation in these runners remains unclear.

IMPLICATIONS OF IRON DEFICIENCY FOR PEDIATRIC POPULATIONS

Although this review is focused on the effects of iron depletion on exercise performance, low body iron stores may have more general implications for health among children and adolescents. Impaired intellectual performance, poor attention span, perceptual problems, and abnormal conduct that interferes with school achievement have been attributed to iron deficiency (Deinard, List, Lindgren, Hunt, & Chang, 1986), although the methodology of studies examining this issue has been questioned (Oski, 1979). Infants with iron deficiency and anemia have a greater incidence of retarded weight gain; the effects of iron depletion in rapidly growing adolescents has not been evaluated. Gastrointestinal abnormalities (gastritis, malabsorption, occult bleeding) and skin and mucous membrane changes (stomatitis, glossitis) are well-documented consequences of iron deficiency.

An association may exist between iron deficiency and susceptibility to infection. Cell-mediated immunity and phagocytosis can be impaired by iron depletion, and there is evidence that iron therapy can reduce the incidence of infection in those who are iron deficient. Conversely, other information suggests there may be a risk of promoting certain bacterial and parasitic infections with iron treatment. Iron is an essential nutrient for pathogenic microbes, and growth of these agents is reduced in an iron-deficient environment. Animal studies have demonstrated that iron treatment increases the severity of several types of bacterial infection, but the relevance of these findings to humans is unclear (Cook & Lynch, 1986).

These data suggest that an increased frequency of iron deficiency in adolescent athletes has broader significance than simply the impairment of exercise performance. The possible impact of iron deficiency on school performance, conduct, and general health should provide a strong stimulus for better understanding the etiology and management of depleted iron stores in these individuals.

MANAGEMENT GUIDELINES FOR IRON DEFICIENCY IN YOUNG ATHLETES

Based on available research information, it is difficult to confidently formulate guidelines for iron supplementation in high school athletes. From laboratory testing, iron deficiency appears to be a significant problem, at least in female adolescent runners among whom approximately 50% will demonstrate low ferritin levels during a competitive season. If this represents true iron depletion, and if nonanemic iron deficiency in fact affects exercise as well as classroom performance, interventions to improve iron stores in these athletes become critically important. Enough evidence exists that either of these conclusions may be invalid, however, thus lending caution to any all-out recommendations for iron therapy. In the absence of more definitive studies, the American Academy of Pediatrics has recommended assessment of iron status for females with "a serious commitment to exercise performance" and males from "low socioeconomic or other backgrounds that may compromise their diet" (Smith, 1983, p. 174).

Counseling athletes to consume diets rich in iron is a commonsense approach to the problem but may not be an effective solution. Because the average diet contains only 5-6 mg of iron per 1,000 kcal, it is difficult to significantly raise iron stores in an individual with overt iron deficiency or ongoing iron losses by diet alone (Clement & Sawchuck, 1984). Still, emphasizing the consumption of foods such as iron-enriched breakfast cereals, poultry, green vegetables, and lean red meat seems prudent.

Routine screening of athletes with determination of serum ferritin levels permits selective iron therapy for those who may be at risk from impaired performance from iron deficiency. Testing for serum ferritin is expensive, however, and may not be readily available in all locations. Ferritin levels fall during training, and only 64% of the 14 high school runners with apparent iron deficiency reported by Rowland et al. (1987) were identified at the start of the season. Effective screening, therefore, requires at least two ferritin determinations (at the beginning and middle) during a competitive season. Anemia is uncommon in high school athletes and, as discussed previously, is a late indicator of iron deficiency. For these reasons, routine measurement of Hb concentration is not recommended as a screening test for iron deficiency.

Should iron supplementation be routinely advised for all endurance athletes in vigorous training regimens? This approach has been advocated for women (Ullyot, 1976) and might be considered when serum ferritin screening is impractical. Others have emphasized that because of the inconclusive evidence for the benefits of iron therapy on exercise performance, routine supplementation is not warranted at the present time (Van Swearingen, 1986). Adverse effects of short-term iron therapy are infrequent and usually minor (constipation, diarrhea, gastric distress). Stools frequently turn black with iron treatment, and some tests for detection of occult stool blood may be invalidated (Herbert, 1965). Oral iron may interfere with gastrointestinal zinc absorption, but the implication for athletes is unknown (Solomons, Pineda, Viteri, & Sandstead, 1983).

CHALLENGES FOR FUTURE RESEARCH

The questions raised by the current limited pool of information on iron deficiency in adolescent athletes deserve close attention. Why does ferritin fall during endurance training? Are individuals with hypoferritinemia and normal Hb concentrations truly iron deficient, and, if so, what are the implications for exercise performance? Is there a threshold of serum ferritin level that indicates physiologically significant iron depletion? Is this phenomenon limited to endurance sports, or does iron status deserve attention in all adolescent athletes? If true iron deficiency is present, what dose of supplementary iron is indicated for competitive athletes?

The possibility of a particular significance of iron deficiency for pediatric athletes needs clarification. Although there is no reason a priori to suspect differences in iron metabolism in this age group compared with adults, the exaggerated needs for iron during the pubertal growth spurt may create a high-risk period for iron deficiency. No information is currently available regarding iron deficiency in prepubertal athletes.

The role of ascorbic acid (vitamin C) in iron deficient athletes merits investigation. Ascorbic acid is important in the reduction of iron from the ferric (Fe^{+3}) to ferrous (Fe^{+2}) state, a process necessary for gastrointestinal absorption as well as for the incorporation of iron into ferritin. A fall in tissue ferritin concentration has been demonstrated in animals deficient in ascorbic acid (Roeser, 1983). Other data suggest a role for ascorbic acid in the enzymatic release of iron from ferritin. Clinical studies on ascorbic acid depletion have shown a parallel fall in maximal aerobic power (Buzina & Suboticanec, 1985). Vitamin C requirements may be increased at times of stress, but supplementary vitamin C has been shown to have no significant effect on exercise performance (Katch & McArdle, 1983).

A greater understanding of the response of serum ferritin to exercise may provide alternative explanations for falling levels with training. For example, binding of ferritin to lymphocytes in the blood may occur under certain conditions such as viral infections (Moroz, Lahat, Biniaminov, & Ramot, 1977). Exercise effects significant changes in lymphocyte subset populations, a situation that could alter serum ferritin concentrations (Berk et al., 1986).

REFERENCES

Alyea, E.P., & Parish, H.H. (1958). Renal response to exercise—Urinary findings. *Journal of the American Medical Association*, **167**, 807-813.

Berk, L.S., Nieman, D., Tan, S.A., Nehlsen-Cannarella, S., Kramer, J., Eby, W.C., & Owens, M. (1986). Lymphocyte subset changes during acute maximal exercise. *Medicine and Science in Sports and Exercise*, **18**, 706.

Blacklock, N.S. (1977). Bladder trauma in the long distance runner. *British Journal of Urology*, **49**, 129-132.

Boileau, M., Fuchs, E., & Barry, J.M. (1980). Stress hematuria: Athletic pseudonephritis in marathoners. *Urology*, **15**, 471-474.

Buckle, R.M., & Cantab, M.D. (1965). Exertional (march) haemoglobinuria:

Reduction of haemolytic episodes by use of sorbo-rubber insoles in shoes. *Lancet*, **1**, 1136-1138.

Buick, F.J., Gledhill, N., Froese, A.B., Spriet, L., & Meyers, E.C. (1980). Effect of induced erythrocytemia on aerobic work capacity. *Journal of Applied Physiology*, **48**, 636-642.

Buzina, R., & Suboticanec, K. (1985). Vitamin C and physical working capacity. *International Journal for Vitamin and Nutrition Research*, **27**, 157-166.

Cantwell, J.D. (1981). Gastrointestinal disorders in runners. *Journal of the American Medical Association*, **246**, 1404-1405.

Carlson, D.L., & Mawdsley, R.H. (1986). Sports anemia: A review of the literature. *American Journal of Sports Medicine*, **14**, 109-112.

Celsing, F., Blomstrand, E., Werner, B., Pihlstedt, P., & Ekblom, B. (1986). Effects of iron deficiency on endurance and muscle enzyme activity in man. *Medicine and Science in Sports and Exercise*, **18**, 151-161.

Clausen, J.P. (1977). Effects of physical training on cardiovascular adjustments to exercise in man. *Physiological Reviews*, **57**, 779-815.

Clement, D.B., & Asmundson, R.C. (1982). Nutritional intake and hematological parameters in endurance runners. *The Physician and Sportsmedicine*, **10**, 37-43.

Clement, D.B., & Sawchuck, L.L. (1984). Iron status and sports performance. *Sportsmedicine*, **1**, 65-74.

Colt, E., & Heyman, B. (1984). Low ferritin levels in runners. *Journal of Sportsmedicine*, **24**, 13-17.

Cook, J.D., Finch, C.A., & Smith, N.J. (1976). Evaluation of the iron status of a population. *Blood*, **48**, 449-455.

Cook, J.D., & Lynch, S.R. (1986). The liabilities of iron deficiency. *Blood*, **68**, 803-809.

Crowell, D.L., Crouse, S.F., Hooper, P.L., & Simon, T.L. (1985). Hematologic parameters in endurance trained and sedentary men (Abstract). *Medicine and Science in Sports and Exercise*, **17**, 293.

Davies, C.T.M. (1974). The physiologic effects of iron deficiency anemia and malnutrition on exercise performance in East African school children. *Acta Paediatrica Belgica*, **28**(Suppl.), 253-256.

Davies, K.J.A., Donovan, C.M., Refino, C.J., Brooks, G.A., Packer, L., & Dallman, P.R. (1984). Distinguishing effects of anemia and muscle iron deficiency on exercise bioenergetics in the rat. *American Journal of Physiology*, **246**, E535-E543.

Davies, K.J.A., Maguire, J.J., Brooks, G.A., Dallman, P.R., & Packer, L.

(1982). Muscle mitochondrial biogenergetics, oxygen supply, and work capacity during dietary iron deficiency and repletion. *American Journal of Physiology,* **242**, E418-E427.

Deinard, A.S., List, A., Lindgren B., Hunt, J.V., & Chang, P.N. (1986). Cognitive deficits in iron-deficient and iron-deficient anemic children. *Journal of Pediatrics,* **108**, 681-689.

Dickson, D.N., Wilkinson, R.L., & Noakes, T.D. (1982). Effects of ultra-marathon training and racing on hematologic parameters and serum ferritin levels in well-trained athletes. *International Journal of Sports Medicine,* **3**, 111-117.

Dressendorfer, R.H., Wade, C.E., & Amsterdam, E.A. (1981). Development of pseudoanemia in marathon runners during a 20-day road race. *Journal of the American Medical Association,* **246**, 1215-1219.

Dufaux, B., Hoedrath, A., Streitberger, I., Hollman, W., & Assmann, G. (1981). Serum ferritin, transferrin, haptoglobin, and iron in middle- and long-distance runners, elite rowers, and professional racing cyclists. *International Journal of Sports Medicine,* **2**, 43-46.

Ehn, L., Carlmark, B., & Hoglund, S. (1980). Iron status in athletes involved in intense physical activity. *Medicine and Science in Sports and Exercise,* **12**, 61-64.

Ericsson, P. (1970). The effect of iron supplementation on the physical work capacity in the elderly. *Acta Medica Scandinavica,* **188**, 361-374.

Falsetti, H.L., Burke, E.R., Feld, R.D., Frederick, E.C., & Ratering, C. (1983). Hematological variations after endurance running with hard- and soft-soled running shoes. *The Physician and Sportsmedicine,* **11**, 118-127.

Finch, C.A., Miller, L.R., Inamdar, A.R., Person, R., Seiler, K., & Mackler, B. (1976). Iron deficiency in the rat. Physiological and biochemical studies of muscle dysfunction. *Journal of Clinical Investigation,* **58**, 447-453.

Frederickson, L.A., Puhl, J.L., & Runyan, W.S. (1983). Effect of training on indices of iron status of young female cross country runners. *Medicine and Science in Sports and Exercise,* **15**, 271-276.

Gilligan, D.R., Altschule, M.D., & Katersky, E.M. (1943). Physiological intravascular hemolysis of exercise: Hemoglobinemia and hemoglobinuria following cross country runs. *Journal of Clinical Investigation,* **22**, 859-869.

Greisen, G. (1986). Mild anemia in African school children: Effect on running performance and an intervention trial. *Acta Paediatrica Scandinavica,* **75**, 662-667.

Haymes, E.M., Puhl, J.L., & Temples, T.E. (1986). Training for cross country skiing and iron status. *Medicine and Science in Sports and Exercise,* **18**, 162-167.

Herbert, V. (1965). Drugs effective in iron deficiency and other hypochromic anemias. In L.S. Goodman & S. Gillman (Eds.), *The pharmacologic basis of therapeutics* (3rd ed., p. 1394). New York: MacMillan.

Jacobs, A., & Worwood, M. (1975). Clinical and biochemical implications. *New England Journal of Medicine, 292,* 951-956.

Katch, F.I., & McArdle, W.D. (1983). *Nutrition, weight control, and exercise* (2nd ed.) Philadelphia: Lea & Febiger.

Lampe, J., Ellefson, M., Slavin, J., Schwartz, S., & Apple, F. (1987). The effect of marathon running on gastrointestinal transit time and fecal blood loss in women runners (Abstract). *Medicine and Science in Sports and Exercise, 19*(Suppl.), 521.

Lampe, J.W., Slavin, J.L., & Apple, F.S. (1986). Effects of moderate iron supplementation on the iron status of runners with low serum ferritin concentrations (Abstract). *Medicine and Science in Sports and Exercise, 18* (Suppl.), 590.

Latner, A.L. (1975). *Clinical biochemistry* (7th ed.). Philadelphia: W.B. Saunders.

Magnusson, B., Hallberg, L., Rossander, L., & Swolin, B. (1984a). Iron metabolism and "sports anemia": 1. A study of several iron parameters in elite runners with differences in iron status. *Acta Media Scandinavica, 216,* 149-155.

Magnusson, B., Hallberg, L., Rossander, L., & Swolin, B. (1984b). Iron metabolism and "sports anemia": 2. A hematological comparison of elite runners and control subjects. *Acta Medica Scandinavica, 216,* 157-164.

Martin, D.E., Vroon, D.H., May, D.F., & Pilbeam, S.P. (1986). Physiological changes in elite male distance runners training for the Olympic Games. *The Physician and Sportsmedicine, 14,* 152-171.

Matter, M., Stittfall, T., Graves, J., Myburgh, K., Adams, B., Jacobs, P., & Noakes, T.D. (1987). The effect of iron and folate therapy on maximal exercise performance in female marathon runners with iron and folate deficiency. *Clinical Science, 72,* 415-422.

McMahon, L.F., Ryan, M.J., Larson, D., & Fisher, R.L. (1984). Occult gastrointestinal blood loss in marathon runners. *Annals of Internal Medicine, 100,* 846-847.

Moroz, C., Lahat, N., Biniaminov, M., & Ramot, B. (1977). Ferritin on the surface of lymphocytes in Hodgkin's disease patients. *Clinical and Experimental Immunology, 29,* 30-35.

Nickerson, H.J., Holubets, M., Tripp, A.D., & Pierce, W.G. (1985). Decreased iron stores in high school female runners. *American Journal of Diseases of Children, 139,* 1115-1119.

Nickerson, H.J., & Tripp, A.D. (1983). Iron deficiency in adolescent cross country runners. *The Physician and Sportsmedicine*, **11**, 60-66.

Ohira, Y., Edgerton, V.R., Gardner, G.W., Senewireatne, B., Barnard, R.J., & Simpson, D.R. (1979). Work capacity, heart rate, and blood lactate responses to iron treatment. *British Journal of Haematology*, **41**, 365-372.

Oski, F.A. (1979). The nonhematologic manifestations of iron deficiency. *American Journal of Diseases of Children*, **133**, 315-322.

Parr, R.B., Bachman, L.A., & Moss, R.A. (1984). Iron deficiency in female athletes. *The Physician and Sportsmedicine*, **12**, 81-86.

Perkkio, M.V., Jansson, L.T., Brooks, G.A., Refino, C.J., & Dallman, P.R. (1985). Work performance in iron deficiency of increasing severity. *Journal of Applied Physiology*, **58**, 1477-1480.

Roeser, H.P. (1983). The role of ascorbic acid in the turnover of storage iron. *Seminars in Hematology*, **20**, 91-100.

Rowland, T.W., Black, S.A., & Kelleher, J.F. (1987). Iron deficiency in adolescent endurance athletes. *Journal of Adolescent Health Care*, **8**, 322-326.

Rowland, T.W., Deisroth, M.A., Green G.M., & Kelleher, J.F. (1987). The effect of iron therapy on the exercise capacity of non-anemic iron deficient adolescent runners. *Medicine and Science in Sports and Exercise*, **19**(Suppl.), S118.

Schoene, R.B., Escourrou, P., Robertson, H.T., Nilson, K.L., Parsons, J.R., & Smith, N.J. (1983). Iron repletion decreases maximal exercise lactate concentrations in female athletes with minimal iron deficiency anemia. *Journal of Laboratory and Clinical Medicine*, **102**, 306-312.

Selby, G.B., & Eichner, E.R. (1986). Endurance swimming, intravascular hemolysis, anemia, and iron depletion. *American Journal of Medicine*, **81**, 791-794.

Siegel, A.J., Hennekens, C.H., Solomon, H.S., & VanBoeckel, B. (1979). Exercise related hematuria, findings in a group of marathon runners. *Journal of the American Medical Association*, **241**, 391-392.

Siimes, M.A., Addiego, J.E., & Dallman, P.R. (1974). Ferritin in serum: Diagnosis of iron deficiency and iron overload in infants and children. *Blood*, **43**, 581-590.

Smith, N.J. (1983). *Sport medicine: Health care for young athletes*. Evanston, IL: American Academy of Pediatrics.

Snyder, A.C., Dvorak, L., & Roepke, J.B. (1987). Dietary pattern and iron parameters of middle aged female runners (Abstract). *Medicine and Science in Sports and Exercise*, **19**(Suppl.), 538.

Solomons, N.W., Pineda, O., Viteri, F., & Sandstead, H.H. (1983). Studies on the bioavailability of zinc in humans: Mechanism of the intestinal interaction of non heme iron and zinc. *Journal of Nutrition*, **113**, 337-349.

Steenkamp, I., Fuller, C., Graves, J., Noakes, T.D., & Jacobs, P. (1986). Marathon running fails to influence RBC survival rates in iron-replete women. *The Physician and Sportsmedicine*, **14**, 89-95.

Stewart, J.G., Ahlquist, D.A., & McGill, D.B. (1984). Gastrointestinal blood loss and anemia in runners. *Annals of Internal Medicine*, **100**, 843-845.

Ullyot, J. (1976). *Women's running*. Mountain View, CA: World Publications.

Van Swearingen, J. (1986). Iron deficiency in athletes: Consequence or adaptation in strenuous activity. *The Journal of Orthopaedic and Sports Physical Therapy*, **7**, 192-195.

Vellar, O.D. (1968). Studies on sweat loss of nutrients: 1. Iron content of whole body sweat and its association with other sweat constituents, serum iron levels, hematological indices, body surface areas, and sweat rate. *Scandinavian Journal of Clinical and Laboratory Investigation*, **21**, 157-167.

Wishnitzer, R., Vorst, E., & Berrebi, A. (1983). Bone marrow depression in competitive distance runners. *International Journal of Sports Medicine*, **4**, 27-30.

Woodson, R.D. (1984). Hemoglobin concentration and exercise capacity. *Annual Review of Respiratory Diseases*, **129**(Suppl.), S72-S75.

Wranne, B., & Woodson, R.D. (1973). A graded treadmill test for rats: Maximal work performance in normal and anemic animals. *Journal of Applied Physiology*, **34**, 732-735.

Wurtman, J.J. (1981). What do children eat? Eating styles of the preschool, elementary school, and adolescent child. In R.M. Suskind (Ed.), *Textbook of pediatric nutrition* (pp. 597-607). New York: Raven.

8

Exercise and the Child With Bronchial Asthma

H.J. Neijens
Erasmus University, Rotterdam

In the majority of asthmatic subjects, exercise has been recognized as an important stimulus for bronchoconstriction. A 5 to 8 min burst of vigorous exercise causes a transient brochodilatation followed by bronchoconstriction, which peaks some 10 to 15 min after completing exercise and may last for up to 1 hr. This is usually called *exercise-induced bronchoconstriction* (EIB), or exercise-induced asthma.

EIB may occur after several types of exercise, although running or cycling are generally the relevant activities in practice. Apart from an early reaction immediately after exercise, a delayed bronchial obstructive reaction has been observed recently, similar to that of antigen-induced bronchial obstruction (Iikura, Inui, Nagakura, & Lee, 1985; Lee, Nagakura, Papageorgiou, Iikura, & Kay, 1983). This late reaction occurs 4 to 24 hr after the completion of exercise. Prolonged early reactions are also occasionally found. Delayed reactions, which may have clinical implications, seem to be observed particularly in children. For example, an apparent spontaneous exacerbation of asthma, especially at night, may be related to exercise undertaken several hours earlier.

191

The prevalence of EIB among asthmatic patients seems to be higher in children than in adults. It has been a clinical impression that EIB gives rise to an important part of the symptoms in asthmatic children, especially those in puberty. Many of these are limited in their daily activities and sports by the occurence of EIB. The occurence of EIB is often determined from a review of the individual's history, or it is ascertained by an exercise test in the laboratory or in the natural setting. It is important to realize that the degree of EIB is influenced by a variety of standardized factors. In the laboratory, exercise can be performed on a treadmill or a cycle ergometer, which allows sufficient intensity to raise heart rate to at least 90% of the age-related maximal level. This load is maintained for 6-8 min. The degree of bronchoconstriction is predominantly expressed as the difference between lung function parameters before and after exercise. If an exercise test is repeated within a couple of hours, the degree of bronchoconstriction after the second test is usually markedly lower than that of the first test. The ability to induce the same amount of bronchoconstriction is mainly recovered after 2 hr and almost always fully within 4 hr (Edmunds, Tooley, & Godfrey, 1978). Thus a refractory period of about 2 to 4 hr exists.

The severity of EIB varies greatly between patients and even in the same patient at different times. An occasional patient develops serious, prolonged, potentially life-threatening attacks of dyspnea, stridor, erythema, itching of the skin, angioedema, gastrointestinal colic, and headache. These attacks are called *exercise-induced anaphylaxis* (Sheffer, Soter, McFadden, & Austen, 1983), which can occur once in a lifetime or repeatedly. EIB has to be discriminated from tachypnea after exercise that is caused by restrictive pulmonary diseases. It is important to recognize the latter abnormalities because those experiencing them are at risk for hypoxia.

VARIABLES IN EXERCISE-INDUCED BRONCHOCONSTRICTION

Amount of Metabolic Stress

Postexercise bronchoconstriction sharply increases with the intensity and duration of exercise. A rise in intensity increases bronchospasm, but no further increase in constriction occurs beyond 60%-85% of the maximal aerobic power (Silverman & Anderson, 1972).

Type of Exercise

Differences in the bronchial response to various kinds of exercise at approximately the same intensity have been reported. Free-range running causes more bronchoconstriction than treadmill running. Cycling was thought to induce a lower drop in lung function than running, whereas walking and swimming were considered even less asthmagenic. Sports such as swimming and kayaking, which focus on arm strength and movement, are less likely to induce bronchial obstruction (Anderson, Conolly, & Godfrey, 1971). These differences in response to exercise were originally thought to be due to the different characteristics of the predominantly used muscle groups. However, several studies have raised doubt about this explanation. If the different types of exercise are carefully matched for metabolic conditions like oxygen consumption, the differneces in EIB disappear (Strauss, Haynes, Ingram, & McFadden, 1977). A linear relationship exists between the metabolic stress as measured by the oxygen consumption during exercise and the muscle mass involved.

Differences in EIB among various sports and among persons of different age and sex diminish markedly when a correction is made for the muscle mass and the amount of ventilation involved. Thus it is likely that the bronchoconstriction that follows different kinds of exercise is largely related to metabolic stress, which is influenced by the amount of the exercise and the muscle mass involved.

Characteristics of Inhaled Air During Exercise

Several observations highlight the importance of the characteristics of the inhaled air in EIB. EIB is more severe when subjects breathe dry air compared to when they breathe humidified air. In patients who develop EIB when breathing with their mouths open, nasal breathing virtually abolishes the postexercise bronchoconstriction (Shturmann-Ellstein, Zeballos, Buckely, & Souhrada, 1978). This may be explained by the humidifying and heating capacity of the nose. An excellent relationship was found between the condition of the inspired air (i.e., temperature and humidity) and the degree of bronchoconstricion after exercise (Deal, McFadden, Ingram, & Jaeger, 1979b). McFadden and Ingram (1979) developed an equation to predict the degree of bronchoconstriction ($\%\Delta$ FEV), from the humidity and temperature of the inspired air and the minute ventilation, which are the components of the respiratory heat exchange (RHE, kcal/min).

$$\%\Delta FEV_1 = 26.10 \cdot RHE - 4.16$$

Strauss, McFadden, Ingram, Deal, and Jaeger (1978) compared temperature and humidity and their interaction with EIB. Heating the air from room to body temperature had no marked effect on the bronchial response. When the humidity was increased in combination with room temperature, the degree of bronchoconstriction diminished. The lung function changes could be completely prevented by fully saturated inhaled air at room temperature.

Eschenbacher and Sheppard (1985) provided convincing evidence that bronchoconstriction provoked by exercise being performed where dry air was inhaled at three separate temperatures (-8.4, 20.5, and 39.4 °C) made little difference to the degree of ensuing bronchoconstriction. Thus it seems that the humidity of the inhaled air is more important than its temperature in causing bronchoconstriction. Temperature may also play a role, however, because a decrease in temperature is associated with a reduction in water content.

Inspired air is know to be heated and humidified so that by the time it approaches the alveoli it is fully saturated with water vapor at body temperature. Heat and water move from the mucosa to the incoming air, as a function of temperature and vapor pressure gradients and the geometric characteristics of the exchanging surface. Heating occurs both by conduction and convection. During air warming, the capacity of air to hold water increases and humidification occurs by evaporation from the airway mucosa.

The net effect of the thermal exchanges on inspiration is to cool and dry the mucosa. This depends upon not only the condition of inspired air and the intensity of ventilation, but also the time of exposure. High levels of ventilation with relatively cold air surpass the warming and humidification capacity of the airways and challenge the deeper airways with cooling and drying. The decrease in temperature in the intrathoracic airways is confirmed by temperature measurements in the retrotracheal part of the esophagus, the magnitude being related to minute ventilation and, inversely, to inspired temperature and water content. A mean temperature of 20 °C in the trachea and 27 °C deep in the right lower lobe is found in healthy subjects inspiring air at -17 °C with moderate hyperventilation (Deal, McFadden, Ingram, & Jaeger, 1979a).

This indicates that very cold air is needed to drop the temperature of the intrathoracic airways with or without modest hyperventilation. However, during pronounced hyperventilation, as in heavy exercise, less cold and dry environmental air may induce bronchial reactions. For the induction of an asthmatic response after exercise, the temperature of inhaled air during pronounced hyperventilation is found to be critical in the range below 20 °C, and the same is true for a water content below 30 mg $H_2O \cdot L^{-1}$. The evidence from most studies points toward the relevance of water loss from the airway mucosa. This concept was extended by Anderson (1984), who showed that, during severe exercise lasting from 6 to 10 min, up to 20 mL water would be required to condition the inspired air to full saturation at 37 °C.

Thus the change in osmolality, rather than the cooling, of the mucosa is the major stimulus for EIB. The expiratory water loss is not different between asthmatic and healthy subjects (Schmidt & Bundgaard, 1986), which suggests that interindividual sensitivity, rather than differences in water loss, determines the bronchial response to exercise. The mechanisms by which an increase in osmolality of the airways could provoke the spread of bronchoconstriction throughout the bronchial tree is still unresolved.

Oxidant air pollution may also play a role, because a concentration of ozone of about 0.20 parts per million was found to be associated with a more pronounced EIB, compared to the reaction in the absence of ozone. Also, the maximal ventilation and ride time were found to be decreased with the presence of ozone (Gong, Bradley, Simmons, & Tashkin, 1986).

Mechanisms of EIB

A number of factors are thought to be important for the bronchial reaction to exercise, including the bronchial mucosa, the mast cells and other cells, the sympathetic and parasympathetic system, and the bronchial smooth muscles.

The presence of increased responses of the bronchi is indicated by the term *bronchial hyperreactivity*. This is a characteristic of asthma and can be quantified by the response of the bronchi to a standardized stimulus, such as inhalation of histamine or metacholine. Bronchial hyperreactivity is related to the presence of asthma and to the severity of the disease. The degree of EIB and the reaction after inhaled histamine appear to be related, indicating that the more pronounced the bronchial reactivity, the greater the EIB. The relationship between the reactions after both stimuli suggests that they develop by similar mechanisms (Bascom & Bleecker, 1986; Neijens, Wesselius, & Kerrebijn, 1981).

Considerable variation may occur in the severity of EIB during the year, with seasonal changes, remissions, and exacerbations in asthmatic symptoms. The variation in EIB is probably related to changes in airway reactivity to histamine or metacholine. The presence of a viral respiratory tract infection or a recent vaccination against influenza may increase the severity of EIB. In sum, any factor that increases the reactivity of the respiratory tree accentuates the response to exercise.

The parts of the bronchial mechanism recognized as contributors to an exaggerated bronchial reaction are the mucosa (increased permeability or sensitivity to physical/chemical changes), the parasympathetic nervous system, mast cells (increased releasability of histamine, leucotrienes, etc.), and possibly others. Information about regulation abnormalities is a prerequisite to discovering possible preventions of EIB.

The change in osmolality, as induced by hyperventilation with dry, cool air, may lead to processes in the airway mucosa. Mucosa cells have the potency to produce bronchoconstricting agents (Lee, Assoufi, Cromwell, & Kay, 1983), which may be relevant to bronchial reactions after exercise. A number of factors point to the role of cells such as mast cells in EIB. Several studies have demonstrated that EIB is associated with an increase in plasma histamine (Anderson et al., 1981) and in neutrophil chemotactic factor (Lee et al., 1984), both of which are mast cell mediators. The levels of these mediators may reach maximum prior to peak bronchoconstriction.

Further evidence for action of mediator release from mast cells is brought about by the induction of meutrophil and monocyte activation. This is shown by an increased expression of complement C36 receptors on circulating neutrophils and monocytes in association with early and late EIB reactions (Papageorgiou et al., 1983). In turn, activation of neutrophils and monocytes may contribute to bronchoconstriction. A mechanism for mast cell activation in EIB has been proposed following the observation that a hyperosmolar environment stimulates histamine secretion from human blood basophils or mast cells dispersed from human lung tissue in an energy-dependent manner (Eggleston, Kagey-Sobotka, Schleimer, & Lichtenstein, 1984).

Flint et al. (1985) demonstrated that human bronchoalveolar mast cells, obtained by lavage, are more sensitive to a hyperosmolar stimulus than mast cells dispersed from human lung parenchyma. This adds support to the hypothesis that an increase in the osmolality of airway mucosa activates mast cells for the secretion of mediators that, in turn, contribute to the airflow obstruction (Lee, 1985). Mediators seem also to be important in the mechanism of the refractory period. O'Byrne and Jones (1986) were able to show that inhibition of prostaglandins by indomethacin could prevent refractoriness after exercise, without altering the constrictive reponse following exercise; however, the precise mechanisms of the refractoriness after EIB are unknown.

Although great strides have been made in increasing our understanding of the mechanism responsible for EIB, many questions remain unanswered. At present it is difficult to explain all the features of EIB on the basis of mast cell activation or of other mediator cells. It is reasonable to assume that EIB is a heterogenous condition of which there are at least two separate pathways leading to the response. The first is the hyperosmolar stimulus to mediator cells. The second is the stimulation of neural reflexes in the airway that might occur both directly from the effect of the hyperosmolar stimulus or indirectly on afferent nerve endings through an interaction of released mediators with sensory nerves. This pathway probably explains the effect of local anesthesia on the oropharynx, which blocks the sensory nerve endings (McNally, Enright, Hirsch, & Souhrada, 1979).

PREVENTION AND TREATMENT

The following actions can be taken at this moment to combat EIB. Based on the information about airway drying and cooling, the patient should try to respire through his or her nose. When the nose is markedly obstructed, the reasons for this disturbance should be examined. Mucosal swelling can often be treated with drugs, whereas anatomical abnormalities such as septum deviations or polyps deserve consideration for surgical correction. The gymnasium halls should have an atmosphere with an optimal temperature and humidity. One can advise an asthmatic patient to increase his or her speed gradually to avoid a pronounced bronchial obstruction and to create a refractory situation, in which intense exercise is permitted without generation of EIB (this is called running through one's asthma). Certain sports are preferable to others when considering the inducibility of EIB. Swimming, wrestling, sprinting, and participating in team sports where running is of short duration are often well tolerated. Cold weather sports, however, are often more difficult to cope with for asthmatics than for healthy children. Downhill skiing, however, is usually tolerable, as are activities in warm and moist air (e.g., swimming).

Proper medication, taken prior to exercise, allows most children with asthma to participate in nearly all sporting events. A number of drugs are effective in the protectin against EIB. The potency of drugs is tested by measuring exercise reaction with and without the adminstration of an agent (Neijens et al., 1981). Atropine and related parasympathetic blocking agents may have a protective effect on EIB, if administered by aerosol. Results vary from no effect to a partial protection. A better protection is usually found after inhalation of disodium cromoglycate (Intal^R). Beta-2-sympathetic agonists are highly effective against EIB in most patients when given by aerosol, whereas oral preparations have variable and less pronunced effects. Xanthine derivatives, such as aminophylline and theophylline, give protection against EIB, depending on their serum levels. For a reasonable result, a theophylline serum level of at least 10 mg $\cdot$ L^{-1} is required. Calcium blockers, which have an established place in the treatment of cardiovascular diseases, possess a slight protective potency. However, future developments resulting in more specific calcium blockers for the bronchi might be of value for EIB. Corticosteroids taken orally or inhaled are of little value in the immediate protection against EIB. However, 2 weeks of treatment with inhaled corticosteroids have also been show to reduce EIB (Hendriksen, 1985). The protective effect of inhaled corticosteroids on EIB is additive upon that achieved with a beta-2-sympathetic agonist (Hendricksen & Dahl, 1983).

A sufficient protection sometimes has to be explored by approximating the optimal dosage for an individual drug or a combination of drugs. The therapeutic effects of drugs on EIB at present can be summarized as follows. Usually, the beta-2-sympathetic agonists are the most effective and parasympathetic antagonists are the least effective. The effect of disodium cromoglycate is intermediate and of sufficient potency in a majority of patients. Because disodium cromoglycate is still without observed side effects after 15 years of experience, it can be considered an important drug for the prevention of bronchial reactions during participation in sports. Many asthmatic children who have EIB can perform sport activities if they administer disodium cromoglycate before the game, which may need repeating after 1 or more hours. If disodium cromoglycate does not produce suffcient protection, the inhalation of a beta-2-sympathetic agonist may be considered, but a too frequent use (arbitrarily, more than two puffs in 4 hr) may result in complications, such as tremor or tachycardia.

For many asthmatic patients, a well-adjusted treatment is the only way to perform daily activities and participate in sports and hence to stay in good physical condition. Several gold medal winners in the Olympic games are asthmatics who were able to reach top levels of performance due to adequate treatment and training.

VALUE OF EXERCISE TRAINING IN ASTHMA

Exercise benefits most children, including those with EIB. Before a child starts a training program, one has to exclude other lung diseases or different disturbances than asthma by clinical examination and appropriate exercise tests. Children with such conditions are at risk for serious complications. Physical training should be tailored to allow children of all physical conditions to exercise according to their abilities.

Several studies have shown that no significant improvement in pulmonary function (Mohsenifar, Horak, Brown, & Koerner, 1983) or mechanical properties of the lung (Casciari, et al., 1981) occurs with training, although maximum exercise ventilation and oxygen consumption improves in most patients (Belman & Mittman, 1980). The effect of training upon EIB in asthmatics is primarily confined to improvement in fitness. Variables such as maximal aerobic power, ventilatory muscle performance, and circulatory adaptations may be modified along with training (Belman & Wasserman, 1981). Psychological encouragement and desensitization of the sensation of dyspnea are probably important contributions to the better physical condition that is often reported as a result of a training program. Sports programs improve general well-being and fitness, which may provide a beneficial effect to an asthmatic subject. Training most likely increases exercise tolerance because of the lower degree of hyperpnea at any level of oxygen consumption or exercise intensity in the fit person. This means that low levels of activity can be performed without distress, and patients may require less medication to control EIB. Thus the patient can avoid EIB and train more vigorously.

CHALLENGES FOR FUTURE RESEARCH

It is important to increase our understanding of the mechanisms by which drying and cooling of the airways leads to bronchoconstriction in suseptible patients. We need to obtain more insight into the structures in the bronchial wall that are responsible for bronchoconstriction due to exercise. Also, it would be worthwhile to unravel the mechanism of the refractory period, which may be based on critical points in the reaction-sequence, determining whether EIB will occur. Insight into the mechanisms of the triggers and the responsible pathways that induce bronchoconstriction, as well as the refractory period, will enable us to design optimal treatment in the future.

REFERENCES

Anderson, S.D. (1984). Is there an unifying hypothesis for exercise-induced asthma? *Journal of Allergy and Clincial Immunology,* **73,** 660-665.

Anderson, S.D., Bye, R.T.P., Schoeffel, R.E., Seale, J.P., Tayler, K.M., & Ferris, L. (1981). Arterial plasma histamine levels at rest, during and after exercise in patients with asthma: Effects of terbutaline aerosol. *Thorax*, **36**, 259-267.

Anderson, S.D. Conolly, N.M., & Godfrey, S. (1971). Comparison of bronchoconstriction induced by cycling and running. *Thorax*, **27**, 718-725.

Bascom, R., & Bleecker, E.R. (1986). Bronchoconstriction induced by distilled water, sensitivity in asthmatics and relationship to exercise-induced bronchospasm. *American Review of Respiratory Diseases*, **134**, 248-253.

Belman, M.J., & Mittman, C. (1980). Ventilatory muscle training improves exercise capacity in chronic obstructive pulmonary disease patients. *American Review of Respiratory Diseases*, **121**, 273-280.

Belman, M.J., & Wasserman, K. (1981). Exercise training and testing in patients with chronic obstructive pulmonary disease. *Basics R.D.*, **10**, 1-6.

Casciari, R.J., Fairshter, R.D., Harrison, A., Morrison, J.J., Blackburn, C., & Wilson, A.F. (1981). Effects of breathing retraining in patients with chronic obstructive pulmonary diseases. *Chest*, **79**, 393-398.

Deal, E.C., Jr., McFadden, E.R., Jr., Ingram, R.H., Jr., & Jaeger, J.J. (1979a). Esophageal temperature during exercise in asthmatic and nonasthmatic subjects. *Journal of Applied Physiology*, **46**, 485-490.

Deal, E.C., Jr., McFadden, E.R., Jr., Ingram, R.H., Jr., & Jaeger, J.J. (1979b) Hyperpnea and heat influx: Initial reaction sequence in exercise-induced asthma. *Journal of Applied Physiology*, **46**, 476-483.

Edmunds, A.T., Tooley, M., & Godfrey, S. (1978). The refractory period after exercise-induced asthma, its duration and relation to the severity of exercise. *American Review of Respiratory Diseases*, **177**, 247-254.

Eggleston, P.A., Kagey-Sobotka, A., Schleimer, R.P., & Lichtenstein, L.M. (1984). Interaction between hyperosmolar and IgE-mediated histamine release from basophils and mast cells. *American Review of Respiratory Diseases*, **130**, 86-91.

Eschenbacher, W.L., & Sheppard, D. (1985). Respiratory heat loss is not the sole stimulus for bronchoconstriction induced by isocapnic hyperpnea with dry air. *American Review of Respiratory Diseases*, **131**, 894-901.

Flint, K.C., Hudspith, B.N., Leung, K.B.P., Pearse, F.L., Brostoff, J., & Johnson, N.M.C.L. (1985). The hyperosmolar release of histamine from bronchoalveolar mast cells and its inhibition by sodium cromoglycate. *Thorax*, **40**, 717.

Gong, H.G., Bradley, P.W., Simmons, M.S., & Tashkin, D.P. (1986). Impaired exercise performance and pulmonary function in elite cyclists during low level ozone exposure in a hot environment. *American Review of Respiratory Diseases*, **134**, 726-733.

Hendriksen, J.M. (1985). Effect of inhalation of corticosteroids on exercise-induced asthma: Randomised double-blind cross-over study of budesonide in asthmatic children. *British Medical Journal*, **291**, 248-249.

Hendriksen, J.M., & Dahl, R. (1983). Effect of inhaled budesonide alone and in combination with low-dose terbutaline in children with exercise-induced asthma. *American Review of Respiratory Diseases*, **128**, 993-997.

Iikura, Y., Inui, H., Nagakura, T., & Lee, T. (1985). Factors predisposing to exercise-induced late asthmatic responses. *Journal of Allergy and Clinical Immunology*, **75**, 285-289.

Lee, T.H. (1985). Heat loss, osmolality and the respiration epithelium. In A.B. Kay (Ed.), *Asthma, clinical pharmacology and therapeutic progress* (pp. 393-400). London: Academic Press.

Lee, T.H., Assoufi, B.K., Cromwell, O., & Kay, A.B. (1983). The link between exercise, respiratory heat exchange and the mast cell in bronchial asthma. *Lancet*, **2**, 164-165.

Lee, T.H., Nagakura, T., Papageorgiou, N., Cromwell, O., Iikura, Y., & Kay, A.B. (1984). Mediators in exercise-induced asthma. *Journal of Allergy and Clincal Immunology*, **73**, 634-639.

Lee, T.H., Nagakura, T., Papageorgiou, T., Iikura, Y., & Kay, A.B. (1983). Exercise-induced late asthmatic reactions with neutrophil chemotactic activity. *New England Journal of Medicine*, **308**, 1502-1505.

McFadden, E.R., Jr., & Ingram, R.H., Jr. (1979). Exercise-induced asthma, observations on the initiating stimulus. *New England Journal of Medicine*, **301**, 763-769.

McNally, F.J., Jr., Enright, P., Hirsch, J.E., & Souhrada, J.H. (1979). The attenuation of exercise-induced bronchoconstriction by oro-pharyngeal anaesthesia. *American Review of Respiratory Diseases*, **119**, 247-252.

Mohsenifar, Z., Horak, D., Brown, H.V., & Koerner, S.K. (1983). Sensitive indices of improvement in a pulmonary rehabilitation program. *Chest*, **83**, 189-192.

Neijens, H.J., Wesselius, T.R., & Kerrebijn, K.F. (1981). Exercise-induced bronchoconstriction as an expression of bronchial hyperreactivity: A study of its mechanism in children. *Thorax*, **36**, 517-522.

O'Byrne, P.M., & Jones, N.L. (1986). The effect of indomethacin on exercise-induced bronchoconstricion and refractoriness after exercise. *American Review of Respiratory Diseases*, **134**, 69-72.

Papageorgiou, N., Carroll, M., Durham, S.R., Lee, T.H., Walsh, G.M., & Kay, A.B. (1983). Complement receptor enhancement as evidence of neutrophil activation following exercise-induced asthma. *Lancet* (**i**), 1220-1223.

Schmidt, A., & Bundgaard, A. (1986). Water loss from the respiratory tract during hyperventilation in normal subjects and in asthmatics. *European Journal of Respiratory Diseases,* **143**(Suppl.), 78-80.

Sheffer, A.L., Soter, N.A., McFadden, E.R., Jr., & Austen, K.F. (1983). Exercise-induced anaphylaxis: A distinct form of physical allergy. *Journal of Allergy and Clinical Immunology,* **71**, 311-316.

Shturmann-Ellstein, R., Zeballos, R.J., Buckely, J.M., & Souhrada, J.F. (1978). The beneficial effect of nasal breathing on exercise-induced bronchoconstriction. *American Review of Respiratory Diseases,* **118**, 65-73.

Silverman, M., & Anderson, S.D. (1972). Standardization of exercise-tests in asthmatic children. *Archives of Diseases in Childhood,* **47**, 882-889.

Strauss, R.H., Haynes, R.L., Ingram, R.H., Jr., & McFadden, E.R., Jr., (1977). Comparison of arm versus leg work in induction of acute episodes of asthma. *Journal of Applied Physiology,* **42**, 565-570.

Strauss, R.H., McFadden, E.R., Jr., Ingram, R.H., Jr., Deal, E.C., Jr., & Jaeger, J.J. (1978). Influence of heat and humidity on the airway obstruction induced by exercise in asthma. *Journal of Clinical Investigation,* **61**, 433-440.

9

Juvenile Hypertension and Exercise

Frederick W. Arensman
Humana Hospital Audobon, Louisville, Kentucky

James L. Christiansen
William B. Strong
Medical College of Georgia, Augusta

The increasing interest in sports and fitness in North America may increase the number of young athletes participating in sporting activities. Even prior to the popularization of jogging and fitness, Michener (1976) estimated that 17 million young Americans participated in organized sports, with 7 million competing in secondary interscholastic activities. If these individuals have blood pressure (BP) distributions similar to those of the normal population (Fixler, Laird, Fitzgerald, Stead, & Adams, 1979), 2%-5% are hypertensive; thus 140,000 to 350,000 youths participating in sport will have elevated blood pressure. These estimates reflect only the young people in organized activities.

Few data are available regarding the prudent management of these young hypertensives. The goals of this chapter are, therefore, to

1. define and classify hypertension by severity in adults, adolescents, and children;

2. discuss exercise-induced hemodynamic changes in normotensive and hypertensive individuals;

3. outline hypertensive children's response to exercise and speculate on the effect of sports and physical activity on the individual with hypertension;

4. delineate evaluation and treatment of hypertension in the young athlete;

5. discuss contraindications to sports participation in the young hypertensive athlete;

6. discuss special consideration in exercise testing of hypertensive children; and

7. define future directions and challenges for research.

DEFINITION OF HYPERTENSION

It is a simple matter to state that hypertension is elevation of BP; it is quite a complex issue to determine how high BP must be before it is abnormal. The National Institutes of Health (NIH, 1987) Second Task Force on Blood Pressure Control in Children recently outlined blood pressure measurements as follows:

1. Normal BP—systolic and diastolic BP less than the 90th percentile for age and sex.

2. High normal BP—systolic and/or diastolic BP greater than or equal to the 90th percentile but less than the 95th percentile for age and sex.

3. Hypertension—systolic and/or diastolic BP greater than or equal to the 95th percentile for age.

4. Severe hypertension—BP measurements persistently greater than the 99th percentile for age and sex.

BP increases with advancing age. Figure 9.1 outlines this normal progression in boys and girls (see also Table 9.1). The clinician must compare an individual patient's BP readings to established norms. BP classification by age is shown in Table 9.1. In addition to age, BP is affected by body habitus. A tall child with weight proportional for age and BP reading greater than the 90th percentile for age *probably* has a normal BP for his or her body habitus. Likewise, obese children with BP measurements greater than the 90th percentile may

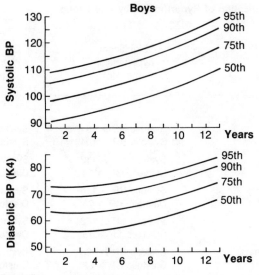

90th Percentile

Systolic BP	105	106	107	108	109	111	112	114	115	117	119	121	124
Diastolic BP	69	68	68	69	69	70	71	73	74	75	76	77	79
Height CM	80	91	100	108	115	122	129	136	141	147	153	159	165
Weight KG	11	14	16	18	22	25	29	34	39	44	50	56	62

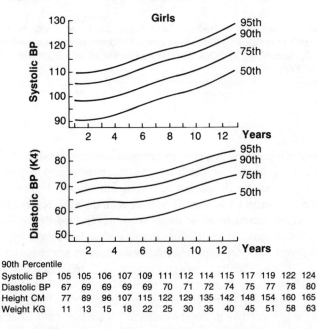

90th Percentile

Systolic BP	105	105	106	107	109	111	112	114	115	117	119	122	124
Diastolic BP	67	69	69	69	69	70	71	72	74	75	77	78	80
Height CM	77	89	96	107	115	122	129	135	142	148	154	160	165
Weight KG	11	13	15	18	22	25	30	35	40	45	51	58	63

Figure 9.1 Age-specific percentiles of BP measurements in 1- to 13-year-old boys and girls. *Note.* From "Report of the Second Task Force on Blood Pressure Control in Children—1987 Task Force on Blood Pressure in Children" by the National Institutes of Health, 1987, *Pediatrics.* REPRODUCED BY PERMISSION OF PEDIATRICS, VOL. 79, PAGE 6, COPYRIGHT 1987.

Table 9.1   Classification of Hypertension by Age Group

Age group	Significant hypertension (mm Hg)	Severe hypertension (mm Hg)
Newborn[a]		
7 days	Systolic BP ⩾ 96	Systolic BP ⩾ 106
8-30 days	Systolic BP ⩾ 104	Systolic BP ⩾ 110
Infant (< 2 years)	Systolic BP ⩾ 112	Systolic BP ⩾ 118
	Diastolic BP ⩾ 74	Diastolic BP ⩾ 82
Children (3-5 years)	Systolic BP ⩾ 116	Systolic BP ⩾ 124
	Diastolic BP ⩾ 76	Diastolic BP ⩾ 84
Children (6-9 years)	Systolic BP ⩾ 122	Systolic BP ⩾ 130
	Diastolic BP ⩾ 78	Diastolic BP ⩾ 86
Children (10-12 years)	Systolic BP ⩾ 126	Systolic BP ⩾ 134
	Diastolic BP ⩾ 82	Diastolic BP ⩾ 90
Adolescents (13-15 years)	Systolic BP ⩾ 136	Systolic BP ⩾ 144
	Diastolic BP ⩾ 86	Diastolic BP ⩾ 92
Adolescents (16-18 years)	Systolic BP ⩾ 142	Systolic BP ⩾ 150
	Diastolic BP ⩾ 92	Diastolic BP ⩾ 98

Note. From "Report of the Second Task Force on Blood Pressure Control in Children—1987 Task Force on Blood Pressure in Children" by the National Institutes of Health, 1987, *Pediatrics*. REPRODUCED BY PERMISSION OF PEDIATRICS, VOL. 79, PAGE 7, COPYRIGHT 1987.
[a]For newborns, only six systolic blood pressures were recorded.

have normal BP for their ponderosity (Prineas, Gillum, Horibe, & Hannan, 1980a). The consideration of lean body mass and ponderosity may be of great importance in assessing the successful young athlete (see Figure 9.2).

A child or adolescent who has BP greater than the 90th percentile for age and who is not particularly tall or heavy requires repeated BP measurements to evaluate for sustained hypertension. In cases other than severe hypertensive crises and severe hypertension, multiple measurements are required to avoid labeling and treating children too aggressively. According to the NIH (1987) report, if BP is greater than or equal to the 90th percentile but there is no end-organ damage or hypertensive crisis, then several closely timed measurements are made according to the algorithm in Figure 9.3. Only after repeated measurements are greater than or equal to the 90th percentile should a youngster be considered as having high normal BP or hypertension.

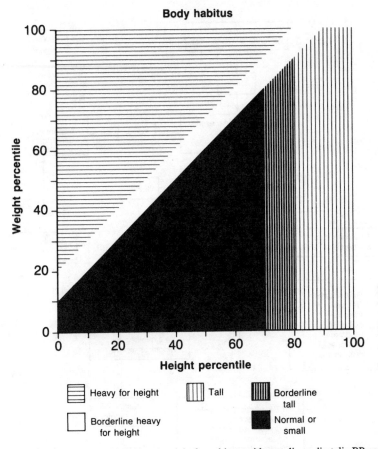

Figure 9.2   Relationship of height and weight for subjects with systolic or diastolic BP greater than or equal to the 90th percentile for age. *Note.* From ''Assessing Children's Blood Pressure—Considerations of Age and Body Size: The Mucatine Study'' by R.M. Lauer, T.L. Burns, & W.R. Clarke, 1985, *Pediatrics.* REPRODUCED BY PERMISSION OF PEDIATRICS, VOL. 75, PAGE 1081, COPYRIGHT 1985.

EXERCISE-INDUCED HEMODYNAMIC CHANGES IN NORMAL INDIVIDUALS

Acute Exercise

Exercise can be divided into dynamic and static components (Schaible & Scheuer, 1985). Dynamic exercise, often referred to as aerobic exercise (although anaerobic exercise can also be dynamic), involves changes in length

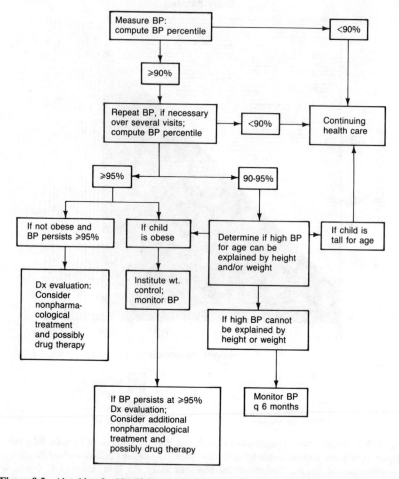

Figure 9.3 Algorithm for identifying children with high BP and initial treatment. *Note.* From "Report of the Second Task Force on Blood Pressure Control in Children—1987 Task Force On Blood Pressure in Children" by the National Institutes of Health, 1987, *Pediatrics.* REPRODUCED BY PERMISSION OF PEDIATRICS, VOL. 79, PAGE 8, COPYRIGHT 1987.

of large muscles and motion of large joints. It usually involves rhythmic contractions of the large muscle groups as in running, rowing, cycling, and swimming.

Static or isometric exercise, by contrast, involves the development of a large force with little or no joint movement and little or no change in muscle length. Objects against which the muscles contract are stationary. Exercises with predominantly isometric components include wrestling, football line blocking, power lifting, the hammer throw, water skiing, and archery. Table 9.2 classifies sports by both level of activity and static and dynamic demands (Mitchell, Blomquist, & Haskell, 1985).

Table 9.2 Classification of Sports

I. Intensity and type of exercise performed
A. High to moderate intensity
1. High to moderate dynamic and static demands
Boxing
Crew/rowing
Cross-country skiing
Cycling
Downhill skiing
Fencing
Football
Ice hockey
Rugby
Running (sprint)
Speed skating
Water polo
Wrestling
2. High to moderate dynamic and low static demands
Badminton
Baseball
Basketball
Field hockey
Lacrosse
Orienteering
Ping-pong
Race walking
Racquetball
Running (distance)
Soccer
Squash
Swimming
Tennis
Volleyball
3. High to moderate static and low dynamic demands
Archery
Auto racing
Diving

Equestrian
Field events (jumping)
Field events (throwing)
Gymnastics
Karate or judo
Motorcycling
Rodeoing
Sailing
Ski jumping
Water skiing
Weight lifting
B. Low intensity (low dynamic and low static demands)
Bowling
Cricket
Curling
Golf
Riflery

II. Danger of body collision
Auto racing*
Bicycling*
Boxing
Diving*
Dowhill skiing*
Equestrian*
Football
Gymnastics*
Ice hockey
Karate or judo
Lacrosse
Motorcycling*
Polo*
Rodeoing*
Rugby
Ski jumping*
Soccer
Water polo*
Water skiing*
Weight lifting*
Wrestling

Note. From "Classification of Sports. A Part of the 16th Bethesda Conference: Cardiovascular Abnormalities in the Athlete: Recommendations Regarding Eligibility for Competition" by J.H. Mitchell, C.G. Blomqvist, & W.L. Haskell. Reprinted with permission from the American College of Cardiology (*Journal of the American College of Cardiology,* **6**(6), 1985, p. 1199.)

*Increased risk if syncope appears.

Both static and dynamic exercise have characteristic cardiovascular responses. Dynamic exercise is accompanied by marked increases in heart rate, cardiac output, and oxygen consumption. The systolic BP increases with increasing intensity of exercise. Diastolic BP remains unchanged, and the mean BP therefore rises (Asmussen, 1981; Schaible & Scheuer, 1985). Systemic vascular resistance can be calculated during exercise using the formula

$$SVR = (MAP - MRAP)/\dot{Q}$$

where SVR is systemic vascular resistance, MAP is mean arterial pressure, MRAP is mean right atrial pressure, and $\dot{Q}$ is cardiac index.

During dynamic exercise, systemic vascular resistance falls because the large increase in cardiac index exceeds the increase in mean arterial pressure. Both heart rate and BP changes are dependent on the exercising muscle group. When oxygen consumption is equal, arm work induces a greater elevation of BP and systemic vascular resistance and a lower cardiac index than work done primarily with the legs (Blomqvist & Saltin, 1983).

By comparison to dynamic exercise, isometric or static exercise is accompanied by relatively smaller increases in oxygen consumption and marked elevation of mean arterial pressure (Nutter, Schlant, & Hurst, 1972). When individuals perform static and then dynamic exercise at the same level of oxygen consumption, the mean BP is shown to rise only with static exercise (Asmussen, 1981).

Intraarterial BPs measured by a catheter during arm curls and leg press weight lifting may be as high as 255/190 and 320/250, respectively (MacDougall, Tuxen, Sale, Moroz, & Sutton, 1985). BP elevation may be secondary to both mechanical compression of the contracting muscle and a pressure reflex of static contraction. Even small muscle mass activation can elicit a sustained elevation in BP. The mass of the contracting muscle appears to be less a factor than the percentage of maximum contraction (Mitchell & Wildenthal, 1974). Systemic vascular resistance remains unchanged when the increase in mean arterial pressure is proportional to the increase in cardiac index. When the mean BP elevation exceeds the increase in cardiac index, the systemic vascular resistance increases. The rise in mean arterial pressure is secondary to elevation in both systolic and, predominantly, diastolic measurements. Diastolic elevation may be secondary to increased cardiac output or the reflex effects originating in the muscles. In addition, during heavy exercise and Valsalva maneuver there is the superimposition of markedly elevated intrathoracic pressure.

Chronic Exercise

Because of the different demands that static and dynamic exercise place on the cardiovascular system, it would be expected that cardiovascular adaptations to chronic static and dynamic exercise may be different. Increased cardiac output accompanying dynamic exercise constitutes a volume overload to the cardiovascular system. The usual adaptive mechanisms to a volume challenge include a large increase in heart rate and a smaller increase in the cardiac stroke volume. Stroke volume is usually augmented by an increased end-diastolic volume and accompanying increased ventricular contraction by the Frank-Starling mechanism.

In contrast to the volume challenge of dynamic exercise, static exercise results in elevated systemic arterial pressures without large increases in the cardiac output. This high intraarterial pressure results in increased left ventricular work and increased myocardial oxygen consumption because of increased ventricular wall tension and increased contractile state (Mitchell et al., 1985). There is little increase in heart rate and only small change in the systolic and diastolic volumes.

Morganroth, Maron, Henry, and Epstein (1975) described echocardiographic similarities and differences between two groups of athletes. They compared endurance athletes (swimmers and runners) to athletes with a major static component in their sport (wrestlers and shot-putters). Increased left ventricular mass was present in both groups. Whereas the swimmers and runners had increased left ventricular internal dimension (increased volume), the wrestlers and shot-putters had increased ventricular thickness of both the interventricular septum and the free ventricular wall. The echocardiographic pattern in the endurance athlete has the appearance of a chronically volume-overloaded heart, whereas the power athlete's heart appears more adapted to high pressure (Schaible & Scheuer, 1985).

No echocardiographic data of which we are aware demonstrate longitudinal changes in a single athlete as he or she undergoes chronic dynamic or isometric training. The cardiac findings in athletes could be the result of genetic predisposition that intrinsically allows better performance with a particular type of activity. These changes in gross cardiac anatomy may mimic those seen in other individuals with abnormal hemodynamics.

Hypertrophy and increased ventricular muscle mass associated with exercise are probably different from hypertrophy associated with chronic pathologic states such as hypertension or aortic stenosis. Left ventricular function is usually normal in the athlete and frequently abnormal in pathologic alterations of hypertension and aortic stenosis. The response to isometric stress is normal in the weight lifter but reduced in the patient with chronic hypertension. A sensitive and potentially early marker for cardiac muscle dysfunction may be diastolic filling changes as measured by Doppler or digitized echocardiography.

Shapiro and McKenna (1984) compared left ventricular diastolic function in swimmers to hypertensive patients with equivalent ventricular hypertrophy. The hypertensive individuals had abnormal function but the swimmers were normal. In a different study, Colan, Sanders, MacPherson, and Borow (1985) compared echocardiographic indexes of diastolic function in swimmers and power lifters to age-matched controls. The hypertrophy in both the swimmers and the power lifters resulted in normal diastolic function. Hypertrophy, per se, may not be the cause of abnormal ventricular filling. Although the athlete's heart sustains only intermittent overload, the ventricle exposed to chronic hypertension or aortic stenosis faces a long-standing pressure overload. The hypertrophy of intermittent pressure overload represents a compensatory adaptation, whereas the hypertrophy associated with constant pressure overload may result in impaired muscle function.

Interesting studies involving spontaneously hypertensive rats have shown the development of myocardial hypertrophy with their hypertension. When they undergo aerobic training, hypertrophy increases, but there may actually be a reversal in abnormalities of the cardiac muscle contractile protein (Rupp & Jacob, 1982; Scheuer, Malhotra, Hirsch, Capasso, & Schaible, 1982).

SPECIAL CONSIDERATIONS IN THE EXERCISE EVALUATION OF HYPERTENSIVE CHILDREN

In pediatric patients there is often an anatomic explanation for hypertension such as coarctation of the aorta. Even after surgery and relief of aortic obstruction, there may be sustained hypertension (see chapter 10 in this book). Beekman, Katz, Moorehead-Steffens, and Rocchini (1983) noted that the baroreceptor response in children was abnormal following relatively late coarctation repair. In a series of six children, the baroreceptor appeared to be reset at a higher baseline and to have diminished sensitivity to changes in arterial pressure. Exercise testing in these children may provide useful information for directing recommendations regarding activities and need for surgical reintervention.

Freed, Rocchini, Rosenthal, Nadas, and Castaneda (1979) demonstrated the efficacy of exercise BPs as a screen for residual postoperative obstruction. They noted a strong correlation between systolic arm pressure and exercise-induced gradient across the site of coarctation. They recommended that exercise BP data guide further investigation such as activity restriction, reoperation, and antihypertensive medication.

Conner (1979) noted that postoperative exercise may generate pressure gradient at the coarctation site that is undetected by routine postoperative evaluation. The increased cardiac output and diminished systemic vascular resistance that accompany exercise may unmask a fixed obstruction at the site of coarctation. The findings at exercise evaluation would include elevated systolic BP in the arms (proximal to the obstruction), fixed BP in the legs (distal to the obstruction), and widening of the arm/leg systolic pressure gradient.

EXERCISE TRAINING IN HYPERTENSION

There seems to be a reduction of rest BP with chronic exercise in both normotensive and hypertensive individuals. A recent critique documents shortcomings of methodology and faults in study design in both cross-sectional and longitudinal experiments (Fagard, M'Buyamba, Staessen, Vanhees, & Amery, 1985). Problems commonly encountered include limitations of age and sex in both control and study populations, small sample size, differences in BP classification among various studies, different methodologies for collection of BP data, and differences in intensity and duration of exercise training programs. Despite these differences, Fagard et al. (1985) concluded that BP reduction with chronic exercise averaged 9 mm systolic and 7 mm diastolic. These relatively small differences indicate that exercise alone cannot replace pharmacologic intervention in individuals with moderate or severe hypertension. In individuals with high normal BP, however, exercise *may* reduce pressures into the normal range.

Kiyonaga, Arakawa, Tanaka, and Shindo (1985) contended that the lack of large reductions in BP with exercise may be secondary to the exercise program's being too strenuous. They reported 12 patients with essential hypertension who trained at 50% of their maximum oxygen consumption by cycle ergometry. The patients had a significant reduction in both systolic and diastolic BPs and effectiveness of training was linked to pretraining plasma renin activity, training-induced reduction in catecholamines, elevation of prostaglandin-E, and increased postexercise urinary excretion of sodium.

Isometric training may also have beneficial effects on rest BP. Six weight-training adolescents were reported by Hagberg et al. (1984), most of whom had undergone previous endurance training. Systolic BP was significantly lower following weight training, and diastolic pressures remained lower in those individuals who had initial diastolic hypertension. When weight training was discontinued, systolic BP rose to preexercise levels and diastolic pressures rose marginally. The authors noted a decrease in systemic vascular resistance during the exercise period of 5 months and stated that weight training may, in some cases, elicit further BP reduction than that expected from endurance training.

The specific cause of BP reduction with chronic exercise is not known, but several theories have been offered (Seals & Hagberg, 1984). Exercise may induce a state of chronic vasodilatation with subsequent reduction in peripheral vascular resistance and BP reduction. A second unproven theory states that hypertension may be the result of a hyperkinetic cardiovascular system. Increased heart rate and increased cardiac output at rest may accompany some forms of hypertension. Chronic exercise may have the beneficial effect of reducing both the heart rate and the cardiac output, via the reduction in sympathetic tone.

Mild exercise may increase prostaglandin-E activity, which may lower BP by its vasodilator effect or enhanced renal sodium excretion (Kiyonaga et al., 1985). In addition, prostaglandin-E may inhibit the release of norepinephrine from nerve terminals, resulting in further reduction in sympathetic tone (Hedqvist, 1970).

THE YOUNG HYPERTENSIVE ATHLETE

Evaluation

The evaluation of the young athlete for hypertension is identical to that of the nonathlete. Hypertension should be defined in childhood as blood pressure exceeding the 95th percentile, confirmed by three measurements on separate occasions. Of all children diagnosed by these criteria, one-third will return to a normal BP when followed over a 3- to 8-year period (Londe, Bourgoignie, Robson, & Goldring, 1971). It is therefore imperative to exercise caution in labeling an individual as hypertensive. The stratification of BP is necessary to establish guidelines for athletic participation. The majority of competitive athletes with hypertension will be adolescents. For this group, adult standards of hypertension may be used (Frohlich, Lowenthal, Miller, Pickering, & Strong, 1985; 16th Bethesda Conference, 1984).

The classification of younger children and preadolescents is more difficult because BP is highly correlated with both height and weight. Some sports emphasize size as a positive attribute to athletic performance; there may, therefore, be a predisposition for successful young athletes to be large and have relatively high BPs. These children who have higher BPs than smaller individuals in their age group may have elevated BPs due to early maturity and growth or large lean body mass (Wilson, Gaffney, Laird, & Fixler, 1985). It is important, therefore, to avoid the overdiagnosis of hypertension in these young athletes. The BP interpretation can be determined by comparison to height and weight rankings so that age alone is not the sole determinant. (See Figure 9.2 for percentile rankings in these incidents.) Another variable is size of the blood pressure cuff. The American Heart Association recommends that the cuff should cover two-thirds of the upper arm, particularly in athletes whose arm circumference may be increased due to large muscle mass. Finally, the athlete's drug regimen should be listed, including nonsteroidal anti-inflammatory drugs, steroids, oral contraceptives, nose drops, and sympathomimetic amines used as nasal decongestants. Less frequently, the athlete may be ingesting amphetamines and/or narcotics. In addition to idiopathic hypertension, the primary care-giver should be aware of a subset of athletes with elevated BP as variant of normal. It is anticipated that patients with an athletic heart syndrome and hyperkinetic heart syndrome fall into this category (Huston, Puffer, & Rodney, 1985). Some athletes have a high resting systolic and a normal diastolic BP (Walther & Tifft, 1985). Little is known regarding the long-term effects of this BP elevation.

Likewise, there is a paucity of data regarding the prevalence and natural history of hypertension in the young athlete. It is well known that high BP is relatively common in football players (Grossman & Baker, 1984; Wilson et al., 1985) and weight lifters (MacDougall et al., 1985). Little is known about the etiology of this hypertension. Confounders may include training methods, lean body mass and maturity, use of exogenous pharmocologic agents, and a natural predisposition for large individuals to compete in these sports. To determine the risk of hypertension in various sports, it is important to recognize that normal athletes may have extreme elevation of BP during certain types of activity (Bryan, 1969). This may be related to the ability to have dramatic increases in cardiac output. Additionally, elevation of arterial pressure has not been observed to be directly related to sudden death during athletic participation. In at least two reviews of pathologic series (Maron, Roberts, McAllister, Rosing, & Epstein, 1980; Virmani, Robinowitz, & McAllister, 1982), hypertension per se has not been implicated as a cause of morbidity or mortality. The long-term effects of athletic participation have not been adequately studied in a longitudinal or epidemiologic manner.

Treatment

The treatment of hypertension in children and adolescents is a subject of debate. As previously stated, at least one-third of children diagnosed as having elevated BP on three isolated occasions will eventually have normal BP without any intervention. We agree with the algorithm as presented by the NIH Task Force (1987; Figure 9.3). Pharmocologic therapy may not be indicated in adolescents with a resting BP of less than 160/95 in the absence of definable etiology. Few data demonstrate ill effects of athletic participation on hypertension or its complications. We therefore suggest that therapy not be initiated in an athlete with mild hypertension who has no evidence of end-organ damage (e.g., retinal lesions or disproportionate left ventricular hypertrophy). Exception to this recognized arbitrary recommendation is the athlete in whom peak BP response to exercise testing is greater than 240 mm of mercury systolic and 95 diastolic. A similar approach is used for isolated resting hypertension of greater than 160/100.

If, on the one hand, the resting systolic BP does not exceed 160, the diastolic pressure is 95 or less, and the exercise systolic BP is less than 240, then our initial approach is to institute hygienic measures. We attempt sodium restriction and weight loss when appropriate. If, on the other hand, resting BP is greater than 160 systolic and the diastolic pressure is equal to or greater than 95, we are more likely to initiate pharmacologic therapy. This course is arbitrarily chosen because 240 mm of mercury exceeds the 95th percentile of BP with exercise.

The goal of therapy is to achieve a normal systolic and resting BP. Occasionally, this goal can be reached exclusively with hygienic measures such as reduction of salt intake, weight loss, and increased levels of aerobic activity. If these methods are unsuccessful and particularly if end-organ damage exists, we advocate pharmacologic intervention. The main thrust of our antihypertensive therapy is somewhat different in the athlete due to the untoward side effects of beta blockers. A major effect of beta blockade is the reduction of maximum heart rate and peak working capacity (Lowenthal et al., 1983). Both of these effects may be poorly tolerated in the high performance athlete. An additional problem in drug therapy involves the use of diuretics in these individuals because of potential fluid and electrolyte abnormalities and the danger of dehydration during long periods of exercise in a hot and/or humid environment.

When pharmacological intervention is initiated, we usually recommended alpha-1 adrenergic inhibition with prazosin. The advantages of this drug include reduction in peripheral vascular resistance without major change in serum lipids, reduction in exercise tolerance, or fluid and electrolyte abnormalities (Kaplan, 1984). In addition, there is a low reported incidence of sexual dysfunction in males taking this medication.

The goal of obtaining normal systolic and diastolic BPs may require additional medications including a diuretic such as thiazide with potassium supplementation or another diazide with potassium-sparing qualities. The schema of intervention at our institution parallels the stepped-care approach as advocated by the Second Task Force of the NIH (1987).

Contraindications to Athletic Participation

Although few data are available regarding the absolute contraindications for participation in sports for the hypertensive athlete, many physicians opt to limit the activity of these young individuals.

The 16th Bethesda Conference (1984) addressed cardiovascular abnormalities in athletes and made recommendations regarding their eligibility for participation. There were suggestions regarding the adult hypertensive participant, but not enough data to warrant recommendations for the adolescent. The task force was divided when polled as to whether hypertensive athletes should be allowed to complete. Numerous reasons were cited for lack of consensus.

At that time, there were not clear guidelines regarding normal BP in adolescents. It was noted that many hypertensive adolescents would become normotensive over time. Additionally, and most convincingly, no data suggested that most competitive aerobic types of sports resulted in any short- or long-term deleterious effects. To avoid the possibility of making these children "cardiac cripples," a prudent course adopted a permissive attitude and allowed participation with reasonably close supervision, such as weekly BP measurements.

Again, hard data are absent, but the 16th Bethesda Conference (1984) recommended unlimited competitive participation in the absence of target organ involvement and severe diastolic ($\geqslant$ 115) hypertension. Its recommendation was to treat adolescents with secondary forms of hypertension or primary hypertension and target organ involvement as adult hypertensives. These individuals could participate in low-intensity competitive sports (Class I.B. in Table 9.2) and should not participate in sports with danger of body collision.

Our Institutions, the Section of Pediatric Cardiology at the Medical College of Georgia and pediatric cardiology at Humana Hospital Audubon, promote and even encourage activity and participation for the following reasons:

1. A program of vigorous dynamic exercise may result in long-term reduction in BP.

2. To the best of our knowledge, no on-field mortality has ever been clearly linked to hypertension (Maron et al., 1980; Strong & Steed, 1982).

3. Intraarterial pressures during weight lifting have been recorded in excess of 400 mm Hg and no documented harm has resulted from these transient elevations. This is not to be taken as an endorsement of that activity or that degree of BP elevation. As a matter of fact, Strong sees no health justification for the sport of power lifting. It confers no health advantages, and repeated frequent BP elevations of that magnitude performed over years to decades may be deleterious to health. When one adds to this stress and the power lifter's frequent abuse of anabolic agents and unusual nutritional supplements, especially amino acid concoctions, one must be highly suspect of the "sport" of power lifting. The statement merely reiterates that high BPs encountered during exercise may not be harmful acutely or chronically.

We concur that follow-up evaluations should be undertaken in these athletes, that a source of the hypertension should be sought, and that the task force recommendation for semiannual or annual visits when athletes attain majority is warranted.

CHALLENGES FOR FUTURE RESEARCH

Few data are available regarding the young hypertensive athlete. Much of the information in this chapter is the result of research on adults. Certainly one must not expect to extrapolate all adult data to childhood problems. Thus, there is a great need for normative data in children. Little is known regarding the natural history of common problems like primary hypertension in childhood. As we become more observant and critical we shall generate information that may aid in prudent and logical management of later hypertensive athletes.

Questions to be addressed include the following:

- What is the incidence of hypertension in a population of young athletes?
- At what level should hypertension be treated?
- What are the advantages of hygienic (nonpharmacologic) treatment in the young athlete?
- What are the long-term benefits and risks of athletic participation for the hypertensive child?

Another exciting challenge may involve the use of exercise testing in normotensive children with a strong family history of hypertension. It has been demonstrated that there is a racial difference in maximum BP response to exercise.

Alpert, Dover, Booker, Martin, and Strong (1961) demonstrated that peak exercise blood pressure was significantly higher in black children than in their white counterparts. Knowing the higher incidence and prevalence of idiopathic hypertension in blacks, one wonders if exercise BP may be a marker for increased cardiovascular reactivity and higher risk for subsequent hypertension.

Our laboratory has performed studies to evaluate exercise BP, cardiac output, and systemic vascular resistance in children at rest and during exercise. Only by long-term follow-up, however, will the predictive value of exercise testing be apparent.

ACKNOWLEDGMENTS

The authors gratefully acknowledge the excellent secretarial assistance of Tonya Gardner and Mary Kamaka.

REFERENCES

Alpert, B.S., Dover, E.V., Booker, D.L., Martin, A.M., & Strong, W.B. (1961). Blood pressure response to dynamic exercise in healthy children—black vs. white. *Journal of Pediatrics,* **99,** 556-561.

Asmussen, E. (1981). Similarities and dissimilarities between static and dynamic exercise. *Circulation Research,* **48**(Suppl. 1), 3-10.

Beekman, R.H., Katz, B.P., Moorehead-Steffens, C, & Rocchini, A.P. (1983). Altered baroreceptor function in children with systolic hypertension after coarctation repair. *American Journal of Cardiology,* **52,** 112-117.

Blomqvist, C.G., & Saltin, B. (1983). Cardiovascular adaptations to physical training. *Annual Review of Physiology,* **45,** 169-189.

Bryan, G.T. (1969). Hypertension in the young athlete. *Texas Medicine,* **65,** 62-65.

Colan, S.D., Sanders, S.P., MacPherson, D., & Borow, K.M. (1985). Left ventricular diastolic function in elite athletes with physiologic cardiac hypertrophy. *Journal of the American College of Cardiology,* **6,** 545-549.

Conner, T.M. (1979). Evaluation of persistent coarctation of aorta after surgery with blood pressure measurement and exercise testing. *American Journal of Cardiology,* **43,** 74-77.

Fagard, R., M'Buyamba, J.R., Staessen, V., Vanhees, L., & Amery, A. (1985). Physical activity and blood pressure. In C.J. Bulpitt (Ed.), *Handbook of hypertension* (pp. 104-130). New York: Elsevier Science.

Fixler, D.E., Laird, W.P., Fitzgerald, V., Stead, S., & Adams, R. (1979). Hypertension screening in schools: Results of the Dallas study. *Pediatrics,* **63,** 32-36.

Freed, M.D., Rocchini, A., Rosenthal, A., Nadas, A.S., Castaneda, A.R. (1979). Exercise-induced hypertension after surgical repair of coarctation of the aorta. *American Journal of Cardiology, 43*, 253-258.

Frohlich, E.D., Lowenthal, D.T., Miller, H.S., Pickering, T., & Strong, W.B. (1985). Task Force: 4. Systemic arterial hypertension. *Journal of the American College of Cardiology, 6*, 1218-1221.

Grossman, M., & Baker, B.E. (1984). Current cardiology problems in sports medicine. *American Journal of Sports Medicine, 12*(4), 262-267.

Hagberg, J.M., Ehsani, A.A., Goldring, D., Hernandez, A., Sinacore, D.R., & Holloszy, J.O. (1984). Effect of weight training on blood pressure and hemodynamics in hypertensive adolescents. *Journal of Pediatrics, 104*, 147-151.

Hedqvist, P. (1970). Studies on the effect of prostaglandin E_1 and E_2 on the sympathetic neuromuscular transmission in some animal tissues. *Acta Physiologica Scandinavica* (Suppl. 345), 1-40.

Huston, T.P., Puffer, J.C., & Rodney, W.M. (1985). The athletic heart syndrome. *New England Journal of Medicine, 313*(1), 24-32.

Kaplan, N.M. (1984). Therapy of mild hypertension: An overview. *American Journal of Cardiology, 53*, 2A-3A.

Kiyonaga, A., Arakawa, K., Tanaka, H., & Shindo, M. (1985). Blood pressure and hormonal responses to aerobic exercise. *Hypertension, 7*, 125-131.

Lauer, R.M., Burns, T.L., & Clarke, W.R. (1985). Assessing children's blood pressure—considerations of age and body size: The Mucatine Study. *Pediatrics, 75*, 1081.

Londe, S., Bourgoignie, J.J., Robson, A.M., Goldring, D. (1971). Hypertension in apparently normal children. *Journal of Pediatrics, 78*, 569.

Lowenthal, D.T., Stein, D., Hare, T.W., Yarnoff, A., Lowenthal, P.J., Saris, S., Falkner, B., & Affrime, M.B. (1983). The clinical pharmacology of cardiovascular drugs during exercise. *Journal of Cardiovascular Rehabilitation, 3*, 829-837.

MacDougall, J.D., Tuxen, D., Sale, D.G., Moroz, J.R., & Sutton, J.R. (1985). Arterial blood pressure response to heavy resistance exercise. *Journal of Applied Physiology, 58*, 785-790.

Maron, B.J., Roberts, W.C., McAllister, H.A., Rosing, D.R., & Epstein, S.E. (1980). Sudden death in young athletes. *Circulation, 62*, 218-229.

Michener, J.A. (1976). *Sports in America.* New York: Random House.

Mitchell, J.H., Blomqvist, C.G., Haskell, W.L. (1985). Classification of sports. A part of the 16th Bethesda Conference: Cardiovascular abnormalities in the athlete: Recommendations regarding eligibility for competition. *Journal of the American College of Cardiology, 6*(6), 1198-1199.

Mitchell, J.H., & Wildenthal, K. (1974). Static isometric exercise and the heart and physiological and clinical considerations. *Annual Review of Medicine,* **325,** 369-381.

Morganroth, J., Maron, B.J., Henry, W.L., & Epstein, S.E. (1975). Comparative left ventricular dimensions in trained athletes. *Annals of Internal Medicine,* **82,** 521-524.

National Institutes of Health. (1987). Report of the second task force on blood pressure control in children—1987 Task Force on Blood Pressure in Children. *Pediatrics,* **79,** 1-25.

Nutter, D.D., Schlant, R.C., & Hurst, J.W. (1972). Isometric exercise and the cardiovascular system. *Modern Concepts of Cardiovascular Disease,* **41,** 11-15.

Prineas, R.J., Gillum, R.F., Horibe, H., & Hannan, P.J. (1980a). Minneapolis children's blood pressure study: 1. Standards of measurements for children's blood pressure. *Hypertension,* **2**(42), I18-I24.

Prineas, R.J., Gillum, R.F., Horibe, H., & Hannan, P.J. (1980b). Minneapolis children's blood pressure study: 2. Multiple determinants of children's blood pressure. *Hypertension,* **2**(42), I24-I28.

Rupp, H., & Jacob, R. (1982). Response of blood pressure and cardiac myosin polymorphism to swimming training in the spontaneously hypertensive rat. *Canadian Journal of Physiology and Pharmacology,* **60,** 1098-1103.

Schaible, T.F., & Scheuer, J. (1985). Cardiac adaptations to chronic exercise. *Progress in Cardiovascular Diseases,* **27,** 297-324.

Scheuer, J., Malhotra, A., Hirsch, C., Capasso, J., & Schaible, T.F. (1982). Physiologic cardiac hypertrophy corrects contractile protein abnormalities associated with pathologic hypertrophy in rats. *Journal of Clinical Investigation,* **70,** 1300-1305.

Seals, D.R. & Hagberg, J.M. (1984). The effect of exercise training on human hypertension: A review. *Medicine and Science in Sports and Exercise,* **16**(3), 207-215.

Shapiro, L.M., & McKenna, W.J. (1984). Left ventricular hypertrophy: Relation of structure to diastolic function in hypertension. *British Heart Journal,* **51,** 637-642.

16th Bethesda Conference (1984). Cardiovascular abnormalities in the athlete: Recommendations regarding eligibility for competition. *Journal of the American College of Cardiology,* **6**(6), 1186-1188.

Strong, W.B., & Steed, D. (1982). Cardiovascular evaluation of the young athlete. *Pediatric Clinics of North America,* **29,** 1325-1339.

Virmani, R., Robinowitz, M., & McAllister, H.A., Jr. (1982). Nontraumatic death in joggers. A series of 30 patients and autopsy. *American Journal of Medicine, 72,* 874-881.

Walther, R.J., & Tifft, C.P. (1985). High blood pressure in the competitive athlete: Guidelines and recommendations. *Physician and Sports Medicine,* **13**(5), 93-114.

Wilson, S.L., Gaffney, F.A., Laird, W.P., & Fixler, D.E. (1985). Body size composition and fitness in adolescents with elevated blood pressures. *Hypertension,* **7**, 417-422.

10

Diagnostic Use of Exercise Testing in Pediatric Cardiology: The Noninvasive Approach

David J. Driscoll
Mayo Medical School, Rochester, Minnesota

The use of exercise testing in pediatric cardiology differs considerably from its use in adult cardiology. In adult cardiology, exercise testing is used primarily to detect a specific pathologic entity: coronary artery occlusive disease and myocardial ischemia. In the assessment of children and adolescents, exercise testing is used infrequently to detect a specific disease process, but it is used to assess the effects of a known disease process or treatment on maximal aerobic power and the cardiorespiratory responses to exercise.

MEASUREMENT OF CARDIOVASCULAR INDICES

Heart Rate and the Electrocardiogram

Heart rate (HR), one of the basic indexes of cardiac response to exercise, is measured from an electrocardiogram (ECG). This can be done manually by averaging several R-to-R intervals. Alternatively, the electrocardiographic signal can be processed through a tachometer, and a direct recording of HR based on each R-to-R interval can be obtained. Many commercially available electrocardiographs are equipped with a tachometer.

The maximal achievable HR during exercise (HRmax) is a useful measurement, but limitations of its usefulness in patients with heart disease must be recognized. Normally, children and adolescents can achieve a HRmax of 190 to 205 beats • min^{-1}, depending on the type of exercise. In adults, however, HRmax declines with increasing age (HRmax = 210 − 0.65 • age). Frequently, whether or not a subject achieves the HRmax for his or her age is used to determine whether the exercise test represents a maximal cardiorespiratory effort. Although this conclusion usually is correct for subjects with a normal cardiovascular system, HRmax cannot be used to assess the level of effort in children with heart disease because many of these patients have chronotropic insufficiency and reduced HRmax. The causes of this chronotropic insufficiency are multifactorial and include alteration in myocardial and sympathetic catecholamine stores and damage to the sinus node and conduction system as a result of cardiac operation (Åstrand & Åstrand, 1958; Crawford, Simpson, & McIlroy, 1967; Daly & Scott, 1959; Driscoll et al., 1984; Eckberg, Drabinsky, & Braunwald, 1971; Ericksson & Bjarke, 1975; Goldstein, Beiser, Stampfer, & Epstein, 1975).

At least three leads of the standard 12-lead ECG should be displayed or recorded continuously during and for 5-10 min after completion of an exercise test. The examiner should have the option of viewing various combinations of leads so that inferior (leads 2, 3, and AVF), anterior right (V1 or V2), and anterior left (V5 or V6) cardiac events can be assessed. In addition, a complete 12-lead ECG should be recorded at rest and at least once during each work load and for several minutes after exercise. Ideally, the electrocardiograph should have several recording speeds. We prefer to record the 12-lead ECG at 50 mm • s^{-1} paper speed to facilitate measurement of ST segment change. In addition, the ECG can be recorded continuously at 5 mm • s^{-1} paper speed for accurate quantitation of arrhythmia.

Appropriate application of the electrocardiographic electrodes, electrocardiographic leads, and electrical shielding of the cable connecting the electrocardiograph to the patient is critical for obtaining artifact-free electrocardiographic recordings. We prefer to cleanse the skin with alcohol and to lightly abrade it with Number 240 emery paper to reduce skin resistance. Most commercially available electrodes are prepackaged with electrode paste, but occasionally no paste is present, and these electrodes should be discarded or paste applied before using them. The wire leads connecting the individual electrodes to the electrocardiograph cable should be secured to the subject's torso to minimize artifact from movement of the leads during exercise. This can be accomplished by loosely wrapping the torso with an elastic bandage or by using a commercially available knit shirt. The presence of significant artifact on the ECG usually indicates a loose lead-to-electrode interface, a poorly applied electrode, or a lack of electrode paste.

Blood Pressure Measurement

Blood pressure (BP) is an essential measurement in evaluating cardiovascular responses to exercise. BP can be measured directly with an indwelling arterial catheter or needle or, more commonly, indirectly with a cuff, a sphygmomanometer, and a stethoscope to determine the Korotkoff sounds. Numerous commercial electronic units are available to indirectly measure BP during exercise; however, one must be concerned about the accuracy and precision of these "black boxes." Devices designed to insufflate and exsufflate the cuff automatically and a microphone that can be attached over the brachial artery and retained in that position during the exercise study are useful. Because the Korotkoff sounds may be difficult to hear, the fifth rather than the fourth sound usually is used to indicate diastolic BP. Several sizes of cuffs should be available to be used on children of different sizes. The bladder of the cuff should completely encircle the arm, and the width of the cuff should be at least two-thirds the length of the upper arm. An oversized cuff should be available to measure leg BP when indicated.

Direct BP measurement allows nearly instantaneous beat-to-beat monitoring with a high level of precision. However, because of peripheral amplification, measurement of BP in the distal vascular system (radial or brachial artery) overestimates central aortic blood pressure (Figure 10.1; Rasmussen et al., 1985). In addition, this technique is invasive and potentially painful, which limits its usefulness in children.

Cardiac Output and Stroke Volume

The two techniques used most frequently to measure cardiac output ($\dot{Q}$) relatively noninvasively and without the need for radioactive material are the CO_2 (Jones & Campbell, 1982) and the acetylene-helium (Triebwasser et al., 1977) rebreathing techniques.

The CO_2 rebreathing technique is based on the relationship

$$\dot{Q} = \dot{V}CO_2 \div (C_{\bar{v}}CO_2 - C_aCO_2)$$

where $\dot{V}CO_2$ is the volume of carbon dioxide, $C_{\bar{v}}CO_2$ is the mixed venous CO_2 content, and C_aCO_2 is the arterial CO_2 content. $\dot{V}CO_2$ is measured. Mixed venous CO_2 content is calculated from the measurement of alveolar PCO_2,

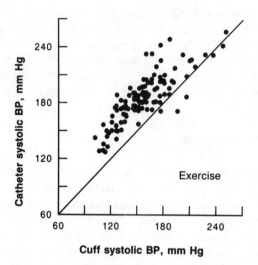

Figure 10.1 Relationship of blood pressure of adolescents and adults determined directly (via radial artery) and indirectly. These data were collected from children, adolescents, and adults. *Note.* From "Direct and Indirect Blood Pressure During Exercise" by P.H. Rasmussen et al., 1985, *Chest,* **87**, p. 743. Copyright 1985 by Chest. Reprinted by permission.

assuming equilibration of mixed venous PCO_2 and alveolar PCO_2 during the rebreathing maneuver. Arterial CO_2 content is calculated from the measurement of arterial PCO_2. The need to measure arterial PCO_2 is a disadvantage of this technique because it is invasive. Arterial PCO_2 can be estimated from end-tidal PCO_2, but this extrapolation introduces an additional source of potential error into the technique. In addition, the concentration of CO_2 in the rebreath mixture, as well as the volume of the rebreath mixture, has to be adjusted to the patient's size and exercise intensity. With considerable experience, however, the CO_2 rebreathing technique can be accurate and useful (Godfrey, 1974).

The acetylene-helium rebreathing technique of measuring $\dot{Q}$ is based on the principle that acetylene diffuses from the alveolus to the pulmonary capillary so that the concentration of acetylene in the rebreath system declines relative to the volume of effective pulmonary blood flow (Figure 10.2). This technique actually measures effective pulmonary blood flow rather than systemic blood flow ($\dot{Q}s$), but, in the absence of significant right-to-left or left-to-right intracardiac or intrapulmonary shunting, it is a reliable approximation of $\dot{Q}s$. In general, however, cardiac output is underestimated by about 7% to 10% using this technique (Smyth, Gledhill, Froese, & Jamnik, 1984). It is necessary to include a gas that does not diffuse out of the alveolus (e.g., helium) to determine the volume of the entire respiratory system and rebreath apparatus. This technique is completely noninvasive and tolerated well by children of all ages (Driscoll et al., 1986). Technically, it is simpler to perform the acetylene-helium rebreath maneuver than the CO_2 rebreath maneuver because the concentration of acetylene, helium, oxygen, and nitrogen used as the rebreath mixture is constant; only the volume of the mixture needs to be altered depending on the subject's size and exercise intensity. Subjects find the acetylene-helium rebreathing technique less uncomfortable (feeling of dyspnea during the rebreath procedure) than the CO_2 rebreathing technique.

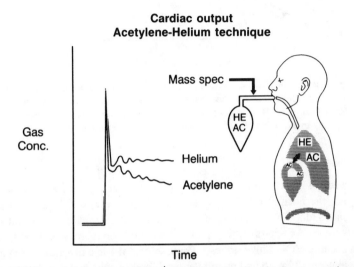

Figure 10.2 Technique of determining $\dot{Q}$. The subject breathes for five to seven breaths from a closed anesthesia bag containing a mixture of O_2, N_2, acetylene, and helium. Gas concentration is measured at the mouthpiece using a mass spectrometer. Acetylene diffuses from the lungs into the pulmonary vasculature. The curves at the left of the figure illustrate the equilibration of helium and the decline of acetylene concentration with each breath.

Doppler echocardiography may be a useful method to assess $\dot{Q}$ and provide nearly instantaneous beat-to-beat measurement of stroke volume and $\dot{Q}$ (Figure 10.3; Ensing, Driscoll, & Tajik, 1986). A Doppler signal is directed into the ascending aorta, usually from the suprasternal notch location. Provided one knows the cross-sectional area of the aorta (obtained by echocardiographic measurements), he or she can approximate stroke volume and $\dot{Q}$.

$\dot{Q}$ is related physiologically to $\dot{V}O_2$:

$$\dot{Q} = \dot{V}O_2/([Hb] \cdot 1.34)(S_aO_2 - S_{\bar{v}}O_2)$$

where [Hb] is the concentration of hemoglobin, S_aO_2 is the arterial blood oxygen saturation, and $S_{\bar{v}}O_2$ is the mixed venous blood oxygen saturation. As can be appreciated, this relationship can be described by regression analysis. For each $1L \cdot min^{-1}$ increase of oxygen consumption, cardiac output should increase

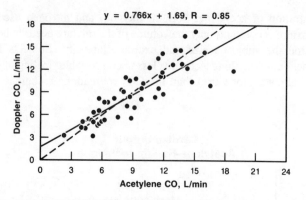

Figure 10.3 Relationship between Q̇ of children, adolescents, and young adults determined by Doppler echocardiography and by acetylene-helium rebreathing technique. (Broken line represents identity.) *Note.* Data from *Measurement of Cardiac Output During Exercise Using Doppler Echocardiography* by G.Ensing, D. Driscoll, and D.J. Tajik, 1986 (unpublished).

approximately 4-4.5 L $\cdot$ min^{-1}. Assuming arterial blood oxygen content remains unchanged, the normal relationship between Q̇ and V̇O_2 can change only if mixed venous blood oxygen content is abnormal (i.e., increased tissue extraction of oxygen). For example, with poor cardiac function, Q̇ may be abnormally low at a specific V̇O_2. This implies, of course, that tissue extraction of oxygen must be abnormally high and mixed venous blood oxygen content abnormally low. Thus, to assess whether Q̇ response to exercise is normal or abnormal, one also must measure V̇O_2 or mixed venous blood oxygen content and compare Q̇ to V̇O_2 or oxygen content of the mixed venous blood. Because V̇O_2 can be measured noninvasively, Q̇ is usually compared to V̇O_2. It is impossible to assess normality or abnormality of Q̇ response to exercise by analyzing Q̇ response alone.

Stroke volume (SV) can be calculated from Q̇ (SV = Q̇ $\div$ HR). Because HR may increase by 1 to 5 beats $\cdot$ min^{-1} during measurement of Q̇ by rebreathing techniques, it is important to measure HR during the rebreathing maneuver to accurately estimate stroke volume.

Blood Oxygen Saturation

Noninvasive (ear or finger oximetry) measurement of blood oxygen saturation can be useful during exercise testing of children with congenital heart disease either to determine and document the presence or absence of hypoxemia or to quantify the degree of hypoxemia. There is an excellent correlation between blood oxygen saturation measured by ear oximetry and that measured by direct blood gas analysis (Figure 10.4). However, at low levels of blood oxygen saturation, this relationship is less precise.

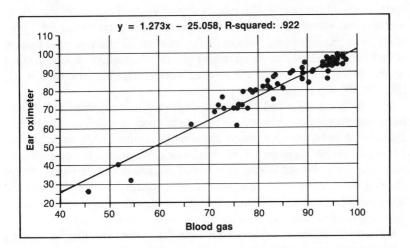

Figure 10.4 Relationship between blood oxygen saturation measured by blood analysis and by ear oximetry for adolescents and adults.

Ventricular Function

Ejection fraction, $\dot{Q}$, and ventricular wall motion abnormalities are measured at rest and during exercise by using radionuclide techniques. However, because this method is invasive and requires injection of a radioactive material, it has limited usefulness for routine exercise testing in children. Its use should be restricted to assessment of specific problems in selected patients.

Echocardographic techniques are useful to assess ventricular function at rest, and some investigators have been successful in adapting this technique for measurements during exercise. Unfortunately, it is technically difficult to obtain echocardiographic measurements during exercise because of movement of the heart within the mediastinum and interposition of pulmonary tissue (an air interface) between the position of the transducer and the cardiac structures.

Ventricular systolic time intervals are determined by phonocardiography and carotid pulse tracing. This is accomplished quite simply at rest and immediately after exercise. However, it is difficult to obtain these measurements during exercise. In addition, because systolic time intervals are affected by HR, contractility, preload, and afterload, their utility as measures of ventricular function is limited (Cokkinos et al., 1985; Moene, Mook, Kruizinga, Bergstra, & Bossina, 1975; Van Der Hoeven, Clevens, Donders, Beneken, & Vonk, 1977).

Ventilatory Measurements

The usefulness of measuring indexes of ventilation during exercise in assessing the response to exercise of patients with cardiac disease is being recognized with increasing frequency. The relationship of ventilation at peak exercise to rest maximal voluntary ventilation may be helpful in determining the degree of effort on the part of the subject during an exercise study and the amount of ventilatory reserve. The measurement of $\dot{V}O_2$ is essential to assess maximal aerobic power and to define the level of work so that measurements of $\dot{Q}$, HR, and BP can be interpreted.

Recently it was suggested that the anaerobic or ventilatory threshold is a useful measurement of maximal aerobic power and a point that defines the optimum exercise intensity for exercise conditioning (Reybrouck, Weymans, Stijns, Knops, & van der Hauwaert, 1985; Reybrouck, Weymans, Stijns, & van der Hauwaert, 1986; Wolfe, Washington, Daberkow, Murphy, & Brammel, 1986). Some authors believe that the anaerobic or ventilatory threshold defines the beginning of lactate accumulation, but other investigators doubt this relationship (for more details, see chapter 5.)

We have found the ventilatory equivalent for oxygen (ventilation ÷ $\dot{V}O_2$) helpful in understanding the limiting factors to exercise in patients with cyanotic congenital heart disease. The oxygen pulse ($\dot{V}O_2$ ÷ HR) has been used as an indicator of stroke volume changes with exercise. However, as can be appreciated from the following relationships, oxygen pulse is dependent on changes in not only stroke volume but also mixed venous oxygen content and arterial blood oxygen content.

$$O_2 \text{ pulse } = \dot{V}O_2 \div HR, \text{ because}$$

$$\dot{V}O_2 = C_aO_2 - C_vO_2,$$
$$\dot{Q} = HR \cdot SV, \text{ and}$$
$$O_2 \text{ pulse } = SV \ (C_a)2 - C_vO_2)$$

where C_aO_2 is the arterial O_2 content and $C_{\bar{v}}O_2$ is the mixed venous O_2 content.

Obviously, if $\dot{Q}$ is measured directly (using CO_2 or acetylene-helium rebreathing techniques), stroke volume is calculated and assessment of O_2 pulse adds little more.

COMMON APPLICATIONS OF EXERCISE TESTING

Exercise testing has been used in assessing a wide variety of cardiac problems in children and adolescents. The clinical usefulness of exercise testing has been documented in many of these situations but is less clear in others. This section discusses clinical situations in which the technique has proven utility. Those situations in which its usefulness requires further study are discussed in the following section.

Measurement of Efficacy of Cardiac Operation

A well-designed exercise test allows not only an objective measurement of the effect of medical treatment or operation but also insight into the mechanisms of change induced by treatment.

Pulmonary Valvotomy.   In 1968, Jonsson and Kee studied 17 adult patients with pulmonary stenosis and noted that maximal aerobic power was normal preopertively as well as postoperatively. They described a reduced cardiac output response to exercise (relative to oxygen uptake), which had also been described by earlier investigators (Johnson, 1962). However, Finnegan, Ihenacho, Singh, and Abrams (1974) found normal cardiac output response in 14 patients after repair of pulmonary stenosis. They speculated that unrelieved persistent pulmonary stenosis and the older ages of patients in previous studies accounted for these observational differences. Stone, Bessinger, Lucas, and Moller (1974) provided a provocative and important study of pulmonary stenosis. These investigators found, as had earlier investigators, that maximum aerobic power was not affected by operation. However, preoperatively in 12 of 20 patients, right ventricular end-diastolic pressure increased with exercise, and in many there was a simultaneous reduction in stroke volume, indicating impaired myocardial function. Postoperatively, no patient had this abnormal response, indicating that abnormal ventricular function was reversible in children by adequate pulmonary valvotomy.

Aortic Valvotomy.   Several hemodynamic changes have been documented during exercise after aortic valvotomy for congenital aortic valve stenosis (Alpert, Kartodihardjo, Harp, Izukawa, & Strong, 1981; Barton, Katz, Schork, & Rosenthal, 1983; Chandramouli, Ehmke, & Lauer, 1975; Cueto & Moller, 1973; James, Schwartz, Kaplan, & Spilkin, 1982; Lee, Jonsson, Bevegård, Karlöf, & Aström, 1970; Orsmond, Bessinger, & Moller, 1980; Whitmer, James, Kaplan, Schwartz, & Sandker Knight, 1981). Maximal aerobic power increased postoperatively, and this improvement was most marked in patients who had moderately severe or severe aortic stenosis preoperatively. Also, maximal systolic blood pressure during exercise was greater postoperatively than preoperatively, and the prevalence of ST segment change during exercise was lower postoperatively than preoperatively.

Repair of Tetralogy of Fallot.   There have been numerous studies of the cardiorespiratory response to exercise after repair of tetralogy of Fallot. James et al. (1976) reported abnormally low maximal aerobic power in 43 patients. Persistently low maximal aerobic power also has been reported by Bjarke (1975); Strieder, Aziz, Zaver, and Fellows (1975); Cumming (1979); Wessel et al. (1980); and Hannon, Danielson, Puga, Heise, and Driscoll (1985). James et al. (1976) found that the reduction in maximal aerobic power was inversely related to age at the time of correction of the cardiac defect, but Hannon et al. (1985; Figure 10.5) and Wessel et al. (1980) did not find this association. The discrepancy probably resulted from studying dissimilar age groups.

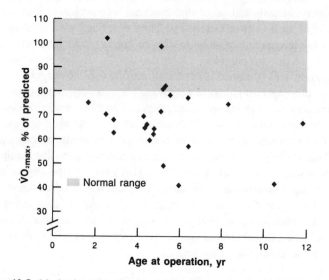

Figure 10.5 Maximal aerobic power in patients after repair of tetralogy of Fallot as related to their age at operation. *Note.* From "Cardiorespiratory Response to Exercise After Repair of Tetralogy of Fallot" by J.D. Hannon, G.K. Danielson, F.J. Puga, C.T. Heise, & D.J. Driscoll, 1985, p. 396. Copyright 1985 by the Texas Heart Institute. Reproduced with permission from the *Texas Heart Institute Journal* (vol. 12, no. 4).

Rocchini (1981) reported reduced cardiac output (when related to oxygen uptake) during exercise after repair of tetralogy of Fallot, and this was also noted by Bjarke (1975), Epstein et al. (1973), and Hannon et al. (1985). It seems reasonable that reduction of maximal aerobic power after repair of tetralogy of Fallot might be related to unrelieved right ventricular outflow tract obstruction or to pulmonary insufficiency. In the study by Wessel et al. (1980), patients with right ventricular pressure greater than 50 mm Hg had more marked exercise intolerance than patients with right ventricular pressure less than 50 mm Hg. However, Hannon et al. (1985) could not document a relationship between maximal aerobic power and right ventricular pressure, the ratio of right ventricular to left ventricular pressure, or the right ventricular to pulmonary artery pressure gradient measured at the end of the operation. Rocchini (1981) found no difference in maximum aerobic power for patients with a transannular patch and pulmonary insufficiency compared to those with a right ventricular-to-pulmonary conduit containing a valve and no pulmonary insufficiency. These discrepancies probably result from studies of groups of patients of dissimilar ages or who had operations at dissimilar ages.

Transposition of the Great Arteries. Mustard's operation is the classic operation for patients with simple d-transposition of the great arteries, in which the aorta arises from the right ventricle and the pulmonary artery from the left ventricle. Systemic venous return is directed by an interatrial baffle through the mitral valve and into the left ventricle. Pulmonary venous return is directed through the tricuspid valve into the right ventricle. The morphologic right ventricle, therefore, must pump against systemic resistance, and the left ventricle is the subpulmonary ventricle. Mathews et al. (1983) studied 21 patients who had had this operation and noted a significantly lower maximal $\dot{V}O_2$ during treadmill exercise in patients (34 ± 7 mL • kg • min^{-1} compared to controls (51.1 ± 10 mL • kg • min^{-1}). Despite their low maximal aerobic power, none of the patients had subjective exercise intolerance. Arrhythmia occurred during or after exercise in 72% of the patients. Abnormal right ventricular function and chronotropic insufficiency contributed to the diminished maximal aerobic power. Several groups of investigators (Benson et al., 1982; Murphy et al., 1983; Parrish et al., 1983; Ramsay, Venables, Kelly, & Kalff, 1984) have studied right ventricular function at rest and during exercise by using radionuclide techniques, and they described either no change or reduced augmentation of right ventricular ejection fraction with exercise in patients who had Mustard's operation. Ensing, Heise, and Driscoll (1988) described abnormal cardiac output response to exercise after Mustard's operation. This was attributed to a combination of reduced or lack of stroke volume increase with exercise and reduced heart rate response to exercise.

Ebstein's Anomaly of the Tricuspid Valve. Ebstein's anomaly of the tricuspid valve consists of an enlarged anterior tricuspid valve leaflet that is adherent to the right ventricular surface and results in an atrialized portion of the right ventricle. The septal leaflet of the tricuspid valve is underdeveloped, and in many cases an atrial septal defect is present. The atrial septal defect allows a right-to-left interatrial shunt and systemic arterial hypoxemia. Surgical repair of this anomaly includes closure of the atrial septal defect and repair or replacement of the tricuspid valve. In a group of 38 patients with Ebstein's anomaly (Barber, Danielson, Heise, & Driscoll, 1985; Driscoll, Mottram, & Danielson, 1988), maximal $\dot{V}O_2$ was only 20.5 ± 7 mL/kg • min^{-1} preoperatively. However, preoperative patients without an atrial septal defect (no right-to-left shunt) had significantly greater maximal $\dot{V}O_2$ (25.3 ± 8 mL• kg^{-1} • min^{-1}) than those with an atrial septal defect (18.9 ± 5 mL• kg^{-1} • min^{-1}). Maximal aerobic power was significantly higher ($\dot{V}O_2 = 26.6 \pm 7$ mL• kg^{-1} • min^{-1}) in a group of 11 postoperative patients. In the preoperative group, systemic arterial blood oxygen saturation was $87.8 \pm 9\%$ at rest and declined to

76.9 ± 15% with exercise. Postoperatively, systemic arterial blood oxygen saturation was normal.

Perhaps the most striking abnormality apparent during exercise in patients with uncorrected cyanotic congenital heart disease is excessive ventilation. The ventilatory equivalent for oxygen was high at rest (48 ± 13 preoperatively vs. 37 ± 6 postoperatively) and during exercise (53 ± 23 vs. 38 ± 6 postoperatively) in the patients with Ebstein's anomaly. The ratio of minute ventilation with exercise to maximum voluntary ventilation at rest was similar preoperatively (50 ± 17%) and postoperatively (52 ± 10%), but this ratio was achieved at a significantly lower mechanical power and $\dot{V}O_2$ for the preoperative than the postoperative group. Ironically, in cyanotic patients with congenital heart disease, maximal aerobic power may be limited by ventilation.

Single Ventricle. The Fontan operation has been applied for about a decade to the repair of tricuspid atresia and other forms of functional single ventricle. The modified Fontan operation results in an unique anatomic and physiologic arrangement. Because there is only one functional ventricle, systemic venous return is directed to the pulmonary artery without the benefit of forward propulsion by a ventricle. The determinants of pulmonary blood flow after the operation are unclear, but pulmonary blood flow probably depends, to a large degree, on ventilatory factors. We (Driscoll et al., 1984; Driscoll et al., 1986) have characterized the cardiorespiratory responses to exercise before and after the Fontan operation. Preoperatively, there is an abnormally low maximal aerobic power ($\dot{V}O_2$max = 43 ± 13.6% of predicted). In addition, maximal aerobic power declined with increasing age at the time of exercise (Figure 10.6). Systemic arterial blood oxygen saturation was low at rest (80%) and during exercise (63%), and the ventilatory equivalent for oxygen was elevated (rest $\dot{V}_E/\dot{V}O_2$ = 59%; exercise $\dot{V}_E/\dot{V}O_2$ = 65%). After operation, maximal aerobic power remained subnormal, but exercise tolerance increased significantly from control values. Similar to the preoperative patients, there was a decline in maximal aerobic power with increasing age at the time of exercise postoperatively. Systemic arterial blood oxygen saturation was increased postoperatively both at rest (94%) and during exercise (92%), but it still was significantly lower than normal, presumably due to small, clinically nonapparent, intrapulmonary right-to-left shunt. Although ventilatory responses to exercise (rest $\dot{V}_E/\dot{V}O_2$ = 56%; exercise $\dot{V}_E/\dot{V}O_2$ = 40%) returned toward normal, ventilation was not completely normal. Postoperatively, $\dot{Q}$ and SV responses were abnormal (Figure 10.7). In addition, HR at peak exercise was reduced (84% of predicted).

The mechanism for abnormal $\dot{Q}$ at rest and during exercise after the Fontan operation probably is related to a systemic ventricle that has been compromised by chronic volume overload and from the lack of a subpulmonary ventricle. Baker, Wilen, Boyd, Dinh, and Franciosa (1984) showed that right ventricular function is an important determinate of maximal oxygen uptake in patients with abnormal left ventricular function. Decreased $\dot{Q}$ and SV responses to exercise occur in patients with chronic congestive heart failure.

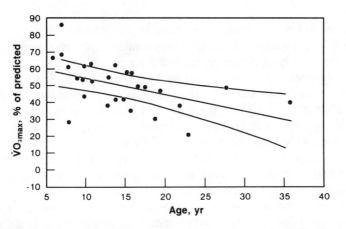

Figure 10.6 Declining aerobic exercise tolerance with increasing age after the Fontan procedure for repair of single ventricle. Lines denote mean and 95% interval for a mean Y value. *Note.* Reprinted with permission of the American College of Cardiology (*Journal of the American College of Cardiology*, Vol. 7; May, 1986; page 1087).

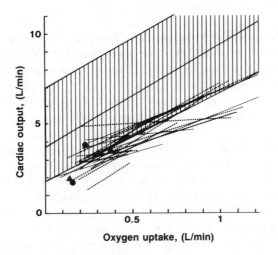

Figure 10.7 Abnormal cardiac output response measured after Fontan operation for single ventricle. Hatched area represents normative range, as obtained in the author's laboratory. *Note.* Reprinted with permission of the American College of Cardiology (*Journal of the American College of Cardiology*, Vol. 7; May, 1986; page 1087).

After the Fontan operation, total systemic vascular resistance remained abnormally elevated during exercise. Because right atrial pressure is abnormally elevated in patients after this operation, systemic arteriolar vascular resistance may not necessarily be as abnormally elevated as is total systemic vascular resistance. However, Weber and Janicki (1985) also demonstrated an abnormal elevation in systemic vascular resistance in patients with chronic congestive heart failure, and the abnormal level of systemic vascular resistance correlated with the severity of congestive heart failure.

It is apparent that ventilation may be the primary limiting factor to exercise for cyanotic patients with functional single ventricle, as noted above for patients with Ebstein's anomaly. The presence of a right-to-left shunt in these patients is a strong stimulus to increase ventilation. However, maintenance of acid-base homeostasis through carbon dioxide elimination probably is a major determinant of the increased ventilation. Because of the right-to-left shunt, only a portion of systemic venous return is exposed to pulmonary gas exchange to allow elimination of carbon dioxide. To maintain near-normal systemic arterial blood partial pressure of carbon dioxide, more carbon dioxide must be removed from the blood reaching the lungs. Indeed, the end-tidal carbon dioxide in patients with a right-to-left shunt is reduced, but arterial PCO_2 is normal or only slightly increased. Increased dead space ventilation and an increase in arterial-alveolar partial pressure of carbon dioxide gradient led Strieder and colleagues (Strieder, Mesko, Zaver, & Gold, 1973; Strieder et al., 1975) to postulate that decreased ability to eliminate carbon dioxide in cyanotic congenital heart disease leads to excessive ventilation.

Pulmonary Atresia With Ventricular Septal Defect.   Pulmonary atresia with ventricular septal defect (PA-VSD) is a complex form of congenital heart disease in which discontinuity of the right ventricle and pulmonary arteries is present. A variable degree of pulmonary artery hypoplasia may occur (Driscoll & McGoon, 1987). Surgical repair of PA-VSD consists of closure of the VSD and establishment of continuity between the right ventricle and the pulmonary artery, usually with a prosthetic conduit containing a valve. If the pulmonary arteries are markedly hypoplastic, the repair must be staged. First, continuity between the right ventricle and pulmonary artery is established, but the VSD is not closed (i.e., *first-stage repair*). Several months later, after pulmonary artery size is increased, the VSD can be closed. Barber, Danielson, Puga, Heise, and Driscoll (1986) studied the cardiorespiratory responses to exercise in 14 patients with PA-VSD prior to operation, 11 after first-stage repair, and 10 after complete repair. Maximal aerobic power increased significantly after the first-stage repair ($\dot{V}O_2$ = 39% [prerepair] and 53% [postrepair] of predicted) but did not increase further after complete repair ($\dot{V}O_2$ = 51% of predicted) and remained significantly less than normal. Systemic arterial blood oxygen saturation increased successively after the first-stage and complete repair (Figure 10.8). After complete repair, $\dot{Q}$ and SV response to exercise remained low relative to oxygen uptake, similar to that observed by Hannon et al. (1985) after repair of tetralogy of Fallot. As noted already with other forms of cyanotic congenital heart disease, ventilation was excessive preoperatively but returned toward normal postoperatively.

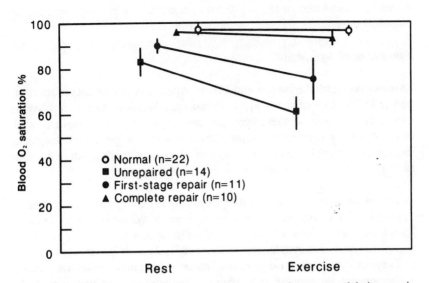

Figure 10.8 Changes in systemic arterial blood oxygen saturation at rest and during exercise before, after first-stage repair, and after complete repair of pulmonary atresia with ventricular septal defect. *Note*. Reprinted with permission of the American College of Cardiology (*Journal of the American College of Cardiology*, Vol. 7; May, 1986; page 630).

Mechanical Pacemaker Systems.   The technology of mechanical pacemaker systems has advanced considerably in the past decade. In contrast to a fixed-rate ventricular demand pacemaker that maintains a predetermined ventricular rate regardless of a patient's level of activity, modern pacemaker systems can adjust the ventricular rate relative to atrial rate (in patients with atrioventricular block) or skeletal muscle activity (activity-activated pacemaker systems). Understandably, if a pacemaker system is designed to change its rate based upon the patient's level of activity, it may be necessary to assess the pacemaker function not only at rest but also during exercise (Bricker et al., 1985). The first step in assessing mechanical pacemaker function is to know specifically what the pacemaker system is programmed to do, based on which the examiner can determine whether or not the unit is functioning satisfactorily.

The availability of variable-rate pacemakers activated by the intrinsic atrial rate or skeletal muscle activity seems to be ideal to allow near normal HR response during exercise for children with complete atrioventricular block or other cardiac abnormalities precluding normal chronotropic response to exercise. Unfortunately, 150 beats • min^{-1} is the practical upper rate limit for most of these pacemaker systems, and when 151 beats • min^{-1} is obtained, the rate decreases abruptly to considerably less than 150 beats • min^{-1}. The abrupt decrease of the ventricular rate usually results in an abrupt cessation of exercise. Technology of mechanical pacemaker systems will continue to improve such that exercise heart rates of 180 to 190 beats • min⁻¹ may be provided for children and adolescents.

Evaluation of Symptoms

Exercise-Associated Syncope and Presyncope. Syncope occurs in approximately 15% to 25% of young people (Boudoulas, Weissler, Lewis, & Warren, 1982). The majority of these syncopal episodes are relatively benign forms of vasodepressor syncope. However, some forms of syncope result from potentially life-threatening conditions, and formal exercise testing can be used to identify some of these conditions.

1. Exercise-associated cardiac arrhythmias are relatively common in patients with repaired congenital heart defects. After the Fontan operation (Driscoll et al., 1986), 38% of patients had an arrhythmia, and after repair of tetralogy of Fallot (Hannon et al., 1985), 25% of patients had an arrhythmia with exercise. Usually, these arrhythmias consist of isolated premature ventricular contractions, couplets, or supraventricular arrhythmias and are unassociated with syncope. However, exercise-induced ventricular tachycardia in a subject with suboptimal cardiac hemodynamics can cause syncope.

2. Catecholamine-sensitive ventricular tachycardia or ventricular fibrillation is a rare, but potentially fatal, phenomenon (Alpert, Boineau, & Strong, 1982; Coumel, Fidelle, Lucet, Attuel, & Bouvrain, 1978). For reasons that are unclear, these patients developed significant ventricular arrhythmia, with increased circulatory levels of catecholamine such as occur with exercise or fright.

3. After abrupt cessation of intense aerobic exercise, Q̇ drops rapidly. If concomitant vasoconstriction does not occur, hypotension and syncope may result. This can be diagnosed by carefully monitoring BP after exercise. Syncope can be avoided by not abruptly stopping exercise but rather using a cool-down period of low-intensity exercise.

4. Exercise testing may be helpful in confirming a diagnosis of hysterical or psychogenic syncope. If the patient has an episode of syncope during a well-monitored exercise test, it can be established that the episode was not due to an arrhythmia or abnormal blood pressure response. Also, observation of the episode may be helpful in establishing its hysterical nature.

5. True cardiac syncope resulting from aortic stenosis, hypertrophic cardiomyopathy, or mitral stenosis is best diagnosed by means other than an exercise test. These conditions should be apparent from clinical examination and other diagnostic procedures.

Chest Pain Syndromes.   Chest pain occurs commonly in children and adolescents. It is usually benign chest-wall pain or costochondritis, and the cause of the pain is apparent from a thorough history and examination. Diagnostic studies usually are not necessary when evaluating these patients (Brenner, Ringel, & Berman, 1984; Coleman, 1984; Driscoll, Glicklich, & Gallen, 1976). However, chest pain, albeit benign, can cause considerable concern for the patient and the parents. They, of course, are concerned that the symptoms may be related to a serious underlying medical problem. Although there have been no well-controlled clinical studies, it has been my impression that much of this undue anxiety and concern can be eliminated by an exercise test. The patient and family will be reassured that no problems occurred, even with the stress of maximum exercise. In this setting, the exercise test is being used as a therapeutic, rather than a diagnostic, tool, and it is important that the family be allowed to observe the test. As noted, however, there has been no scientific assessment to determine whether or not undue anxiety and concern actually are eliminated. Furthermore, use of exercise testing in this fashion should be limited to those situations in which the clinician perceives persistent anxiety and concern.

Rarely, chest pain in children and adolescents can result from a serious underlying problem, and exercise testing may be helpful in elucidating the cause of the pain. Anginal chest pain can result from one of several congenital or acquired coronary artery abnormalities: congenital membranous webs of the coronary ostia, congenital stenosis of the coronary ostia, anomalous origin of the left coronary artery, left anterior descending or circumflex coronary artery from the right coronary artery or right sinus of Valsalva and passage of the anomalous vessel between the aorta and pulmonary artery, and coronary artery obstruction resulting from Kawasaki syndrome. In these instances, which admittedly are rare, exercise may produce ST segment change on the exercise ECG. However, a negative exercise study does not exclude these diagnostic possibilities.

Intermittent cardiac arrhythmia may be interpreted by a child as chest pain, and exercise testing may be helpful in precipitating the arrhythmia.

Aortic Valve Stenosis.   With the advent of Doppler echocardiography, the severity of aortic stenosis (AS) can be estimated noninvasively. However, prior to the clinical application of this technique, investigators attempted to assess the severity of AS with the exercise test, and certain relationships were described between the cardiac responses to exercise and the severity of AS (Alpert et al., 1981; Barton et al., 1983; Chandramouli et al., 1975; Cueto & Moller, 1973; James et al., 1982; Lee et al., 1970; Orsmond et al., 1980; Whitmer et al., 1981). Whitmer et al. (1981) demonstrated an inverse relationship between total work performed and the transaortic pressure gradient: Patients with severe AS had less maximal aerobic power than patients with milder forms of AS. Peak exercise systolic blood pressure was lower for patients with moderate and moderately severe AS than normal control subjects or patients with mild AS. In addition, the degree of ST segment depression increased with increasing severity of AS. Chandramouli et al. (1975) also demonstrated a relationship between the number of millivolts of ST segment depression and the aortic valve gradient. In an elegant study, Kveselis et al. (1985) demonstrated that ST segment change occurring in patients with AS was determined by left ventricular oxygen supply/demand ratios, as estimated by systolic and diastolic pressure-time indexes. Although maximal aerobic power, ST segment change, and BP response during exercise correlated with the severity of AS in a large group of patients, exercise testing was not as helpful, as one might desire, for determining the severity of AS for an individual patient. This, together with the advent of echocardiography and Doppler techniques, has changed the role of exercise testing in patients with AS.

Exercise testing remains useful in evaluating children and adolescents with AS in the following circumstances:

1. There is a small subset of patients with AS who, by pressure gradient criteria, have mild or only moderately severe AS but develop ST segment depression with exercise. One surmises that these patients have disadvantageous left ventricular oxygen supply/demand ratios with exercise and might benefit from aortic valvotomy despite a transaortic pressure gradient that seemingly falls within an acceptable range. One must remember, however, that in postoperative cardiac patients, ST segment change may not be as reliable an indication of altered myocardial oxygen supply/demand ratios as in unoperated patients.

2. Exercise testing may help reassure the physician and patient that exercise and perhaps competitive athletics are safe in a specific patient with mild AS or when an operation brings good results.

3. Exercise testing also may be helpful in determining whether or not chest pain in a patient with AS is a result of myocardial ischemia secondary to the valvular disease or, in fact, is benign chest wall pain.

Maximal Aerobic Power in Children With Diseases or Malformations. Parents usually overestimate the maximal aerobic power of their children, especially if the child has a disease or malformation. Formal exercise testing allows an objective measurement of maximal aerobic power. Such a measurement may be useful in several circumstances when managing children and adolescents with heart problems.

1. It is useful in reassuring patients with certain relatively minor forms of heart disease that it is safe to exercise. Examples of such forms of heart disease include mitral valve prolapse, bicuspid but unobstructed aortic valve, small ventricular septal defects (VSDs) or repaired VSDs or atrial septal defects with normal pulmonary artery pressure, and well-repaired coarctation of the aorta without hypertension.

2. Knowledge of a patient's maximal aerobic power is useful in counseling patients with significant cardiac abnormalities regarding types of physical activities in which they can engage comfortably and safely. This may be pertinent particularly for children with congenital heart disease who wish to participate in organized athletics. Obviously, it would be futile and frustrating for a child to participate in competitive sports if a cardiac defect severely limited his or her exercise tolerance.

3. A knowledge of the subject's maximal aerobic power is important in designing physical fitness rehabilitation programs and monitoring progress of those programs.

POSSIBLE CLINICAL APPLICATIONS OF EXERCISE TESTING

Coarctation of the Aorta.   Coarctation of the aorta was one of the first forms of congenital heart disease to be repaired surgically. There have been many published reports of the utility of exercise testing to assess the results of this operation and the presence or absence of recurrent or persistent coarctation of the aorta. Unfortunately, the interpretation of the results of these studies still is controversial and, at times, conflicting. Upper level extremity BP can be measured accurately at rest and during exercise. Unfortunately, simultaneous noninvasive measurement of upper and lower extremity BP to determine a pressure gradient across the area of repaired coarctation is nearly impossible. Most investigators have relied on leg BP measurements obtained within 1 min of cessation of exercise. Considering, however, that the decrease of BP on cessation of exercise is variable and can be very abrupt, the interpretation of postexercise leg BP is difficult, perhaps impossible. Also, much confusion exists because there isn't uniform agreement on what constitutes significant recurrent or persistent coarctation of the aorta.

Upper extremity hypertension can persist after apparent successful relief of coarctation of the aorta. Waldman, Goodman, Tumeu, Lambert, and Turner (1980) studied 28 postoperative patients and found that the absence of a rest arm-to-leg BP gradient did not necessarily indicate adequate relief of coarctation. Freed, Rocchini, Rosenthal, Nadas, and Castaneda (1979) reported the results of exercise tests of 30 postoperative patients. Higher upper extremity systolic BP occurred in the postoperative group than in the control group. The mean arm-to-leg BP gradient was 69 mm Hg after exercise, and there was a correlation between systolic BP during exercise and the arm-to-leg BP gradient measured within 1 min of cessation of exercise. There was a correlation between rest and postexercise arm-to-leg BP gradient. They found no correlation between exercise arm systolic BP and age at operation. Connor (1979) performed exercise tests on 13 postoperative patients and concluded that a postexercise arm-to-leg BP gradient of 35 mm Hg or more was an indication for angiography to determine the presence or absence of anatomic obstruction.

Markel et al. (1986) investigated the differences between arm exercise and treadmill leg exercise in patients after repair of coarctation of the aorta. These investigators concluded that upper extremity hypertension during treadmill exercise was due to a marked increase in descending aortic blood flow with mild-to-moderate recurrent or persistent coarctation. Furthermore, they concluded that, on the one hand, patients with a rest arm-to-leg BP gradient greater than 15 mm Hg who developed a large (degree unspecified) arm-to-leg BP gradient after exercise likely have significant persistent or recurrent coarctation. On the other hand, patients with minimal rest arm-to-leg BP gradients, even if upper extremity BP during exercise is above 200 mm Hg, probably do not have significant persistent or recoarctation. Recently, Daniels, James, Loggie, and Kaplan (1987) reported that height, preoperative systolic BP, and residual postoperative arm-to-leg BP gradient were the best correlates of postoperative rest and maximal exercise systolic BP.

The story is confusing. Much of the confusion stems from a lack of understanding of what constitutes important persistent or recurrent coarctation of the aorta and what the indications are for reoperation. In view of this, it is not surprising that the utility of exercise testing in assessing the results of coarctation repair is unclear. The following points, however, are probably accurate:

1. The presence of normal upper extremity systolic BP response to exercise in a patient with little or no rest arm-to-leg BP gradient is consistent with an adequately repaired coarctation of the aorta.

2. Rest and/or exercise systolic hypertension can occur in the absence of significant persistent or recurrent coarctation of the aorta.

3. Significant persistent or recurrent coarctation of the aorta can be present despite normal upper extremity BP at rest.

4. Postexercise arm-to-leg BP gradient must be interpreted with caution because of (a) variations in the rate of decrease of BP after exercise and (b) technical difficulties in measuring leg BP.

In summary, exercise testing is a useful clinical tool in assessing patients after repair of coarctation of the aorta and understanding the pathophysiology of this lesion. However, clinical decisions regarding the presence or absence of significant persistent or recurrent coarctation of the aorta should not be made on the basis of the results of the exercise test alone.

Arrhythmias.   Exercise testing may offer insight into the mechanisms and treatment of some cardiac arrhythmias. As already noted, exercise-associated syncope can result from a cardiac arrhythmia, and exercise electrocardiography may allow documentation of this.

Garson, Gillette, Gutgesell, and McNamara (1980) suggested that all patients who have had tetralogy of Fallot repaired should have exercise testing to detect the presence of complex ventricular arrhythmias that could potentially explain the relatively high incidence of sudden death in patients after repair of tetralogy of Fallot. However, one must be cautious not to overinterpret the meaning of ventricular ectopy, which, of course, occurs in normal subjects.

Exercise electrocardiography has been used to study patients with congenital complete atrioventricular block (Karpawich et al., 1981). There are conflicting reports of whether or not the maximal ventricular rate during exercise correlates with the location of block above, within, or below the bundle of His, but it is likely that there is little correlation. Winkler, Freed, and Nadas (1980) observed the presence of ventricular ectopy during exercise in adolescents with congenital complete heart block. Although it has been suggested that this may be an indication for treatment with a mechanical pacemaker, this is still a controversial and unproven point.

It is unclear whether or not exercise testing is a reliable provocative test for arrhythmia, especially for assessment of efficacy of pharmacologic suppression of arrhythmia (Monarrez, Strong, & Rees, 1978; Rozanski, Dimich, Steinfeld, & Kupersmith, 1979). Because the presence of arrhythmia is quite unpredictable, further research in this area is necessary.

Pectus Excavatum.   Considerable confusion exists about the effect, if any, of pectus excavatum on cardiorespiratory function at rest and during exercise. More importantly, researchers disagree about whether or not repair of pectus excavatum has a significant effect on cardiorespiratory function at rest or during exercise. A number of investigators have reported minor abnormalities of rest pulmonary function (reduced vital capacity and total lung capacity) consistent with reduced lung volume or chest wall restriction, or both (Orzalesi & Cook, 1965; Polgar & Koop, 1963). However, these abnormalities are subtle and, in most patients, of questionable clinical importance. Abnormal SV response during upright exercise has been reported in patients with pectus excavatum, but this has not been corroborated by other investigators (Bevegård, 1962). In our laboratory, SV increases normally with exercise in patients with pectus excavatum (Wynn et al., 1988). Also, there has been a report of improvement in maximal oxygen consumption, exercise time, and maximal voluntary ventilation after operation for pectus excavatum (Cahill, Lees, & Robertson, 1984; Puhlson, Cahill, & Robertson, 1987). However, a control group was not studied. In an ongoing study at the Mayo Clinic, investigators have found no significant effect of operation for pectus excavatum on maximal aerobic power compared to a control group of patients with pectus excavatum who have not had operations (Wynn et al., 1988).

Exercise testing is a useful tool to measure maximal aerobic power and cardiorespiratory response to exercise in patients with pectus excavatum. However, it is important to control for increase in body size and to use control groups to accurately interpret the effect of an operation. Except in very unusual cases, repair of pectus excavatum is a cosmetic procedure that does not significantly affect cardiorespiratory response to exercise.

CHALLENGES FOR FUTURE RESEARCH

Improved Noninvasive Assessment of Cardiac Function

Measurement of Cardiac Output and Stroke Volume. Presently non-invasive measurement of cardiac output and stroke volume is performed utilizing acetylene helium or CO_2 rebreathing techniques. Both these techniques measure cardiac output over a period of several heartbeats. Utilizing Doppler technology, noninvasive measurements can be made of stroke volume and cardiac output on a cardiac beat-to-beat basis. This information, once the techniques are perfected and validated, will provide important and interesting understanding of beat-to-beat changes in cardiac function at the beginning of and during exercise.

Measurement of Cardiac Valvular Gradients. Little is known about the implications of changes of transaortic, transpulmonary or transmitral valvular gradients during exercise. It is known that all of these gradients increase as cardiac output increases. However, it is difficult and cumbersome to measure these gradients during exercise using presently amiable invasive techniques. With increased experience and validation of Doppler technology, these gradients can be measured during exercise and this information will offer additional insight into the pathophysiology of these cardiac lesions.

Ventricular Function. At present, nuclear medicine techniques are utilized to assess ventricular function during exercise. Hopefully, with improved echocardiographic technology, myocardial function can be measured during exercise without injecting radioactive substances.

Pediatric Exercise Rehabilitation Programs

Cardiac rehabilitation programs for adults are well established. There have been several studies of the utility of rehabilitation programs for children with congenital heart disease. All of these studies have shown that aerobic capacity can be increased in children with congenital heart disease using an aerobic training program. What has not been demonstrated is whether this increased aerobic capacity persists several years after the training program and whether or not children maintain habits of aerobic activity following a training program.

Physiologic Rate Response of Pacemakers

At present, the upper rate limit of rate response of pacemakers in children is approximately 150-160 beats per minute. This, of course, is inconsistent with an optimum hemodynamic response to exercise. Hopefully, in the future, pacemaker systems can be redesigned such that children will be able to achieve an activity triggered paced heart rate close to 200 beats per minute.

Exercise Protocols

There are several reasons why a continuously increasing workload ("ramp" protocol) would be advantageous for use in clinical exercise testing for children. In the near future several ergometers will be marketed that can facilitate this type of protocol for exercise testing in children.

REFERENCES

Alpert, B.S., Boineau, J., & Strong, W.B. (1982). Exercise-induced ventricular tachycardia. *Pediatric Cardiology,* **2**, 51-55.

Alpert, B.S., Kartodihardjo, W., Harp, R., Izukawa, T., & Strong, W.B. (1981). Exercise blood pressure response: A predictor of severity of aortic stenosis in children. *Journal of Pediatrics,* **98**, 763-765.

Åstrand, P.-O., & Åstrand, I. (1958). Heart rate during muscular work in man exposed to prolonged hypoxia. *Journal of Applied Physiology,* **13**, 75-80.

Baker, B.J., Wilen, M.M., Boyd, C.M., Dinh, H., & Franciosa, J.A. (1984). Relation of right ventricular ejection fraction to exercise capacity in chronic left ventricular failure. *American Journal of Cardiology,* **54**, 596-599.

Barber, G., Danielson, G.K., Heise, C.T., & Driscoll, D.J. (1985). Cardiorespiratory response to exercise in Ebstein's anomaly. *American Journal of Cardiology,* **56**, 509-514.

Barber, G., Danielson, G., Puga, F., Heise, C., & Driscoll, D. (1986). Coronary atresia with ventricular septal defect: Preoperative and postoperative response to exercise. *Journal of the American College of Cardiology,* **7**, 630-638.

Barton, C.W., Katz, B., Schork, M.A., & Rosenthal, A. (1983). Value of treadmill exercise test in pre- and postoperative children with valvular aortic stenosis. *Clinical Cardiology,* **6**, 473-477.

Benson, L.N., Bonet, J., McLaughlin, P., Olley, P.M., Feiglin, D., Druck, M., Trusler, G., Rowe, R.D., & Morch, J. (1982). Assessment of right ventricular function during supine bicycle exercise after Mustard's operation. *Circulation,* **65**, 1052-1059.

Bevegård, S. (1962). Postural circulatory changes at rest and during exercise in patients with funnel chest, with special reference to factors affecting the stroke volume. *Acta Medica Scandinavica,* **171**, 695-713.

Bjarke, B. (1975). Oxygen uptake and cardiac output during submaximal and maximal exercise in adult subjects with totally corrected tetralogy of Fallot. *Acta Medica Scandinavica,* **197**, 177-186.

Boudoulas, H., Weissler, A., Lewis, R., & Warren, J. (1982). The clinical diagnosis of syncope. In W.P. Harvey (Ed.), *Current problems in cardiology*, (Vol. 7, p. 8). Chicago: Yearbook Medical Publishers.

Brenner, J.I., Ringel, R.E., & Berman, M.A. (1984). Cardiologic perspectives of chest pain in childhood: A referral problem? To whom? *Pediatric Clinics of North America*, **31**, 1241-1258.

Bricker, J.T., Garson, A., Jr., Traweek, M.A., Smith, R.T., Ward, K.A., Vargo, T.A., & Gillette, P.C. (1985). The use of exercise testing in children to evaluate abnormalities of pacemaker function not apparent at rest. *Pace*, **8**, 656-660.

Cahill, J., Lees, G., & Robertson, H. (1984). A summary of preoperative and postoperative cardiorespiratory performance in patients undergoing pectus excavatium and cavinatium repair. *Journal of Pediatric Surgery*, **19**, 430-433.

Chandramouli, B., Ehmke, D.A., & Lauer, R.M. (1975). Exercise-induced electrocardiographic changes in children with congenital aortic stenosis. *Journal of Pediatrics*, **87**, 725-730.

Cokkinos, D., DePuey, G., Rivas, A., Castro, C., Burdine, J., Leachman, R., & Hall, R. (1985). Correlations of systolic time intervals and radionuclide angiography at rest and during exercise. *American Heart Journal*, **109**, 104-112.

Coleman, W.L. (1984). Recurrent chest pain in children. *Pediatric Clinics of North America*, **31**, 1007-1026.

Connor, T.M. (1979). Evaluation of persistent coarctation of aorta after surgery with blood pressure measurement and exercise testing. *American Journal of Cardiology*, **43**, 74-78.

Coumel, P., Fidelle, J., Lucet, V., Attuel, P., & Bouvrain, Y. (1978). Catecholamine-induced severe ventricular arrhythmias with Adams-Stokes syndrome in children: Report of four cases. *British Heart Journal*, **40**, 28-37.

Crawford, D.W., Simpson, E., & McIlroy, M.B. (1967). Cardiopulmonary function in Fallot's tetralogy after palliative shunting operations. *American Heart Journal*, **74**, 463-472.

Cueto, L., & Moller, J.H. (1973). Haemodynamics of exercise in children with isolated aortic valvular disease. *British Heart Journal*, **35**, 93-98.

Cumming, G.R. (1979). Maximal supine exercise haemodynamics after open heart surgery for Fallot's tetralogy. *British Heart Journal*, **41**, 683-691.

Daly, M., & Scott, M.J. (1959). The effect of hypoxia on the heart rate of the dog with special reference to the contribution of the carotid body chemoreceptors. *Journal of Physiology* (Cambridge), **145**, 440-446.

Daniels, S., James, F., Loggie, J., & Kaplan, S. (1987). Correlates of resting and maximal exercise systolic blood pressure after repair of coarctation of the aorta: A multivariable analysis. *American Heart Journal*, **113**, 349-353.

Driscoll, D.J., Danielson, G.K., Puga, F.J., Schaff, H.V., Heise, C.T., & Staats, B.A. (1986). Exercise tolerance and cardiorespiratory response to exercise after the Fontan operation for tricuspid atresia or functional single ventricle. *Journal of the American College of Cardiology, 7*, 1087-1094.

Driscoll, D.J., Glicklich, L.B., & Gallen, W.J. (1976). Chest pain in children: A prospective study. *Pediatrics, 57*, 648-651.

Driscoll, D., & McGoon, D. (1987). Pulmonary atresia with ventricular septal defect. In R. Brandenberg, V. Fuster, E. Giuliani, & D. McGoon (Eds.), *Cardiology: Fundamentals and principles* (pp. 1474-1479). Chicago: Yearbook Medical Publishers.

Driscoll, D., Mottram, C., & Danielson, G. (1988). Spectrum of exercise intolerance in 45 patients with Ebstein's anomaly and observations on exercise tolerance in 11 patients after surgical repair. *Journal of the American College of Cardiology, 11*, 831-836.

Driscoll, D.J., Staats, B.A., Heise, C.T., Rice, M., Puga, F., Danielson, G., & Ritter, D. (1984). Functional single ventricle: Cardiorespiratory response to exercise. *Journal of the American College of Cardiology, 4*, 337-342.

Eckberg, D.L. Drabinsky, M., & Braunwald, E. (1971). Defective cardiac parasympathetic control in patients with heart disease. *New England Journal of Medicine, 285*, 877-883.

Ensing, G., Driscoll, D., & Tajik, D.J. (1986). [Measurement of cardiac output during exercise using Doppler echocardiography]. Unpublished raw data.

Ensing, G., Heise, C., & Driscoll, D. (1988). Cardiovascular response to exercise after the Mustard operation for simple and complex transposition of the great vessels. *American Journal of Cardiology, 62*, 617-622.

Epstein, S.E., Beiser, G.D., Goldstein, R.E., Rosing, D.R., Redwood, D.R., & Morrow, A.G. (1973). Hemodynamic abnormalities in response to mild and intense upright exercise following operative correction of an atrial septal defect or tetralogy of Fallot. *Circulation, 47*, 1065-1075.

Eriksson, B.O., & Bjarke, B. (1975). Oxygen uptake, arterial blood gases and blood lactate concentration during submaximal and maximal exercise in adult subjects with shunt-operated tetralogy of Fallot. *Acta Medica Scandinavica, 197*, 187-193.

Finnegan, P., Ihenacho, H.N.C., Singh, S.P., & Abrams, L.D. (1974). Haemodynamic studies at rest and during exercise in pulmonary stenosis after surgery. *British Heart Journal, 36*, 913-918.

Freed, M.D., Rocchini, A., Rosenthal, A., Nadas, A.S., & Castaneda, A.R. (1979). Exercise-induced hypertension after surgical repair of coarctation of the aorta. *American Journal of Cardiology, 43*, 253-258.

Garson, A., Jr., Gillette, P.C., Gutgesell, H.P., & McNamara, D.G. (1980). Stress-induced ventricular arrhythmia after repair of tetralogy of Fallot. *American Journal of Cardiology, 46*, 1006-1012.

Godfrey, S. (1974). *Exercise testing in children*. Philadelphia: W.B. Saunders.

Goldstein, R.E., Beiser, G.D., Stampfer, M., & Epstein, S.E. (1975). Impairment of autonomically mediated heart rate control in patients with cardiac dysfunction. *Circulation Research, 36*, 571-578.

Hannon, J.D., Danielson, G.K., Puga, F.J., Heise, C.T., & Driscoll, D.J. (1985). Cardiorespiratory response to exercise after repair of tetralogy of Fallot. *Texas Heart Institute Journal, 12*, 393-400.

James, F.W., Kaplan, S., Schwartz, D.C., Chou, T.C., Sandker, M.J., & Naylor, V. (1976). Response to exercise in patients after total surgical correction of tetralogy of Fallot. *Circulation, 54*, 671-679.

James, F.W., Schwartz, D.C., Kaplan, S., & Spilkin, S.P. (1982). Exercise electrocardiogram, blood pressure, and working capacity in young patients with valvular or discrete subvalvular aortic stenosis. *American Journal of Cardiology, 50*, 769-775.

Johnson, A.M. (1962). Impaired exercise response and other residue of pulmonary stenosis after valvotomy. *British Heart Journal, 24*, 375-388.

Jones, N., & Campbell, E. (1982). *Clinical exercise testing*. Philadelphia: W.B. Saunders.

Jonsson, B., & Kee, S.J.K. (1968). Haemodynamic effects of exercise in isolated pulmonary stenosis before and after surgery. *British Heart Journal, 30*, 60-66.

Karpawich, P.P., Gillette, P.C., Garson, A., Jr., Hesslein, P.S., Porter, C.B., & McNamara, D.G. (1981). Congenital complete atrioventricular block: Clinical and electrophysiologic predictors of need for pacemaker insertion. *American Journal of Cardiology, 48*, 1098-1102.

Kveselis, D.A., Rocchini, A.P., Rosenthal, A., Crowley, D.C., Dick, M., Snider, R., & Moorehead, C. (1985). Hemodynamic determinants of exercise-induced ST-segment depression in children with valvular aortic stenosis. *American Journal of Cardiology, 55*, 1133-1139.

Lee, S.J.K., Jonsson, B., Bevegård, S., Karlöf, I., & Aström, H. (1970). Hemodynamic changes at rest and during exercise in patients with aortic stenosis of varying severity. *American Heart Journal, 79*, 318-331.

Markel, H., Rocchini, A.P., Beekman, R.H., Martin, J., Palmisano, J., Moorehead, C., & Rosenthal, A. (1986). Exercise-induced hypertension after repair of coarctation of the aorta: Arm versus leg exercise. *Journal of the American College of Cardiology, 8*, 165-171.

Mathews, R.A., Fricker, F.J., Beerman, L.B., Stephenson, R.J., Fischer, D.R., Neches, W.H., Park, S.C., Lenox, C.C., & Zuberbuhler, J.R. (1983). Exercise studies after the Mustard operation in transposition of the great arteries. *American Journal of Cardiology, 51*, 1526-1529.

Moene, R., Mook, G., Kruizinga, K., Bergstra, A., & Bossina, K. (1975). Valve of systolic time intervals in assessing severity of congenital aortic stenosis in children. *British Heart Journal, 37*, 1113-1122.

Monarrez, C.N., Strong, W.B., & Rees, A.H. (1978). Exercise electrocardiography in the evaluation of cardiac dysrhythmias in children. *Paediatrician, 7*, 116-125.

Murphy, J.H., Barlai-Kovach, M.M., Mathews, R.A., Beerman, L.B., Park, S.C., Neches, W.H., & Zuberbuhler, J.R. (1983). Rest and exercise right and left ventricular function late after the Mustard operation: Assessment by radionuclide ventriculography. *American Journal of Cardiology, 51*, 1520-1526.

Orsmond, G.S., Bessinger, F.B., & Moller, J.H. (1980). Rest and exercise hemodynamics in children before and after aortic valvotomy. *American Heart Journal, 99*, 76-86.

Orzalesi, M.M., & Cook, C.D. (1965). Pulmonary function in children with pectus excavatum. *Journal of Pediatrics, 66*, 898-900.

Parrish, M.D., Graham, T.P., Jr., Bender, H.W., Jones, J.P., Patton, J., & Partain, L. (1983). Radionuclide angiographic evaluation of right and left ventricular function during exercise after repair of transposition of the great arteries. Comparison with normal subjects and patients with congenitally corrected transposition. *Circulation, 67*, 178-183.

Polgar, G., & Koop, C.E. (1963). Pulmonary function in pectus excavatum. *Pediatrics, 32*, 209-215.

Puhlson, E., Cahill, J., & Robertson, T. (1987, May). *The value of exercise testing in prediction of improvement following correction of chest wall deformities in children.* Paper presented at the scientific session of the American Pediatric Surgical Association, Hilton Head, SC.

Ramsay, J.M., Venables, A.W., Kelly, M.J., & Kalff, V. (1984). Right and left ventricular function at rest and with exercise after the Mustard operation for transposition of the great arteries. *British Heart Journal, 51*, 364-370.

Rasmussen, P.H., Staats, B.A., Driscoll, D.J., Beck, K.C., Bonekat, H.W., & Wilcox, W.D. (1985). Direct and indirect blood pressure during exercise. *Chest, 87*, 743-748.

Reybrouck, T., Weymans, M., Stijns, H., Knops, J., & van der Hauwaert, L. (1985). Ventilatory anaerobic threshold in healthy children. Age and sex differences. *European Journal of Applied Physiology and Occupational Physiology, 54*, 278-284.

Reybrouck, T., Weymans, M., Stijns, H., & van der Hauwaert, L. (1986). Ventilatory anaerobic threshold for evaluating exercise performance in children with congenital left-to-right intracardiac shunt. *Pediatric Cardiology, 7*, 19-24.

Rocchini, A.P. (1981). Hemodynamic abnormalities in response to supine exercise in patients after operative correction of tetrad of Fallot after early childhood. *American Journal of Cardiology*, **48**, 325-330.

Rozanski, J.J., Dimich, I., Steinfeld, L., & Kupersmith, J. (1979). Maximal exercise stress testing in evaluation of arrhythmias in children: Results and reproducibility. *American Journal of Cardiology*, **43**, 951-956.

Smyth, R., Gledhill, N., Froese, A., & Jamnik, V. (1984). Validation of non-invasive maximal cardiac output measurement. *Medicine and Science in Sports and Exercise*, **16**, 512-515.

Stone, F.M., Bessinger, F.B., Lucas, R.V., & Moller, J.H. (1974). Pre- and postoperative rest and exercise hemodynamics in children with pulmonary stenosis. *Circulation*, **49**, 1102-1106.

Strieder, D.J., Aziz, K., Zaver, A.G., & Fellows, K.E. (1975). Exercise tolerance after repair of tetralogy of Fallot. *Annals of Thoracic Surgery*, **19**, 397-405.

Strieder, D.J., Mesko, Z.G., Zaver, A.G., & Gold, W.M. (1973). Exercise tolerance in chronic hypoxemia due to right-to-left shunt. *Journal of Applied Physiology*, **34**, 853-858.

Triebwasser, J.H., Johnson, R.L., Jr., Burpo, R.P., Campbell, J.C., Reardon, W.C., & Blomqvist, C.G. (1977). Noninvasive determination of cardiac output by a modified acetylene rebreathing procedure utilizing mass spectrometer measurements. *Aviation Space and Environmental Medicine*, **48**, 203-209.

Van Der Hoeven, G., Clevens, P., Donders, J., Beneken, J., & Vonk, J. (1977). A study of systolic time intervals during uninterrupted exercise. *British Heart Journal*, **39**, 242-254.

Waldman, J., Goodman, A., Tumeu, A., Lambert, J., & Turner, S. (1980). Coarctation of the aorta, noninvasive physiological assessment in infants and children before and after operation. *Journal of Thoracic Cardiovascular Surgery*, **80**, 187-197.

Weber, K., & Janicki, J. (1985). Cardiopulmonary exercise testing for evaluation of chronic cardiac failure. *American Journal of Cardiology*, **55**, 22-31A.

Wessel, H.U., Cunningham, W.J., Paul, M.H., Bastanier, C.K., Muster, A.J., & Idriss, F.S. (1980). Exercise performance in tetralogy of Fallot after intracardiac repair. *Journal of Thoracic Cardiovascular Surgery*, **80**, 582-593.

Whitmer, J.T., James, F.W., Kaplan, S., Schwartz, D.C., & Sandker Knight, M.J. (1981). Exercise testing in children before and after surgical treatment of aortic stenosis. *Circulation*, **63**, 254-263.

Winkler, R., Freed, M., & Nadas, A. (1980). Exercise-induced ventricular ectopy in children and young adults with complete heart block. *American Heart Journal*, **99**, 87-92.

Wolfe, R.R., Washington, R., Daberkow, E., Murphy, J.R., & Brammel, H.L. (1986). Anaerobic threshold as a predictor of athletic performance in prepubertal female runners. *American Journal of Diseases of Children*, **140**, 922.

Wynn, S., Ostrum, N., Driscoll, D., O'Connell, E., Telander, R., & Staats, B. (1988). [Exercise tolerance before and after operation for pectus excavatum]. Unpublished raw data.